C.K. Labalen, DDS

SHOW ME YOUR TEETH

FROM MENTAL TO DENTAL

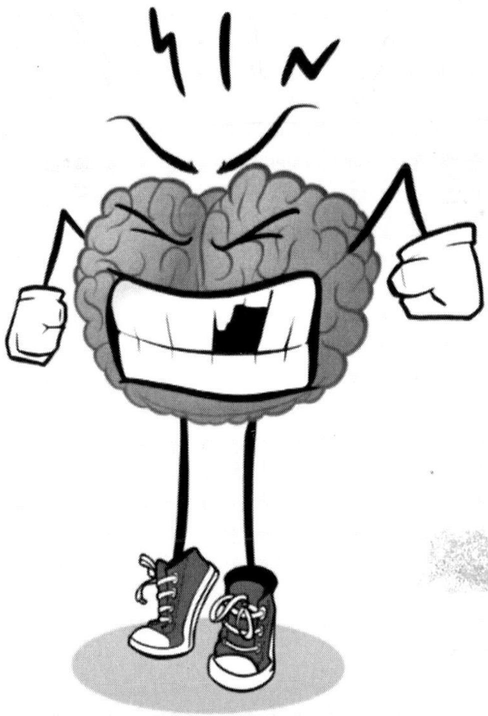

Go to the dentist and smile like you mean it

Printed in the United States of America
First edition, June 2020
ISBN - 978-1-7353178-0-9
www.mental2dental.com

DISCLAIMER

The content of this book is for informational purposes only and is not intended to diagnose, treat, cure, or prevent any condition or disease. It is not intended as a substitute for consultation with a licensed practitioner. Please consult with your dentist regarding the suggestions and recommendations made in this book. The advice we offer with regard to looking for the right practitioner will probably help but choosing a healthcare professional is ultimately the responsibility of the patient.

The publisher and the author make no guarantees concerning the level of success you may experience by following the advice and strategies contained in this book, and results will differ for each individual. The author is a licensed dentist and, as such, is using over thirty years of experience and expertise to help you take responsibility for your oral health.

Ultimately, the choice of professionals is yours, and the quality and responsibility of the treatment belong to them. None of these responsibilities can be transferred to the author or publisher of this book.

Using the information in this book is at your own risk and implies your acceptance of this disclaimer.

Table of Contents

To Alex

"Being deeply loved by someone gives you strength while loving someone deeply gives you courage."
– Lao Tzu

To my parents and siblings

FOREWORD

There are several reasons why I am incredibly pleased to write the foreword to this text. First, to introduce you to a nonconformist in a world of stereotypes and followers. I am a dentist who, for years, has been writing about the confusion in dentistry over a subject called occlusion. It is said to be the most crucial subject in dentistry, yet no one has succeeded in presenting a logical explanation as to why it is confusing. It is so complicated it is not taught in dental schools. A few years back, I received an e-mail from a dentist, Dr. C.K. Labalen, who had recently opened a beautiful, state of the art dental office in a European capital. Not only was this a bold move for a woman to introduce her professional skills to a predominately male area, she offered them classes in postgraduate education. I think most would be intimidated by such a venture, but Dr. Labalen had a free mind and the courage to express it. In her classes, she presented the latest technology in modern dentistry; periodontology, implantology, extractions, surgery, and prosthetic replacements---all except one---occlusion. There was no consensus, only opinions. What was she to teach? A mutual friend and colleague suggested that she contact me as I had written several articles about the difficulties in understanding this important subject. She e-mailed me to obtain my lecture schedule, and I told her that I had no lecture schedule, just an opinion about why this subject defied easy comprehension. I told her, however, that if we could meet, I would spend time with her and explain everything I understood about the subject. Within ten days, Dr. Labalen was sitting in my office in San Francisco, and we spent two days discussing the difficulties in understanding and presenting this vital subject. As in Casablanca, it was the beginning of a beautiful friendship. What kind of person travels six thousand miles to hear someone's opinion?

Dr. Labalen, a graduate of Université de Nice-Sophia Antipolis, is also a freelance writer and publisher. When Spain's economy suffered its deepest recession in half a century, Caroline, rather than fret about her financial status, sought the need to provide benevolent treatment and assistance to those in need for moral and altruistic reasons. She founded an international NGO-Non-Profit whose goal was to develop a structure of clinics that would bring oral health to deprived areas in Tanzania where 23 million people lack primary dental treatment.

Caroline has a genuine love for dentistry. She is one of those exceptional people we are privileged to meet. Her text, Show Me Your Teeth, is a thorough, honest explanation of what every patient needs to understand about maintaining their oral health. It is not just an explanation of what a gold crown is or why you should have your teeth cleaned regularly, but about the obligation of each individual to take responsibility for their dental care. It's about the need to analyze your own problems and make decisions about your treatment. It's about relationships with your health care provider, not selecting a dentist because he/she has a great personality or is attractive, but about finding a dentist who has kindness, empathy, and compassion. It's a must-read.

Gene McCoy D.D.S.
San Francisco, May 2020

ACKNOWLEDGMENTS

I want to thank my three mentors, by order of appearance in my life: Prof. Marc Bolla, who took me from the dental cradle into professional adulthood and taught me the essence of whom I became as a dentist. The late Dr. Carl E. Misch, who guided me for over fifteen years in the world of implantology, giving me the push to be among the best, and showing me how to remain at that level of excellence. You are deeply missed. Dr. Gene McCoy, samurai of occlusion, the base of the pyramid sustaining oral health. His dedication to the profession continues to be an example to follow, and his friendship is a sacred jewel I carry with me. Thanks to Alex and Angie for their help in the first draft, the re-draft, and the re-re-draft of this book. Their patience and support have undoubtedly placed them on the road to angelhood. Thanks to my friends for their relentless and unconditional support and thank you José Rulos for the immense talent and sense of humor you have poured into the book's cover and illustrations. Thanks to Jeffrey Armstrong for showing me the way. Without him, this book would not have seen the light of day.

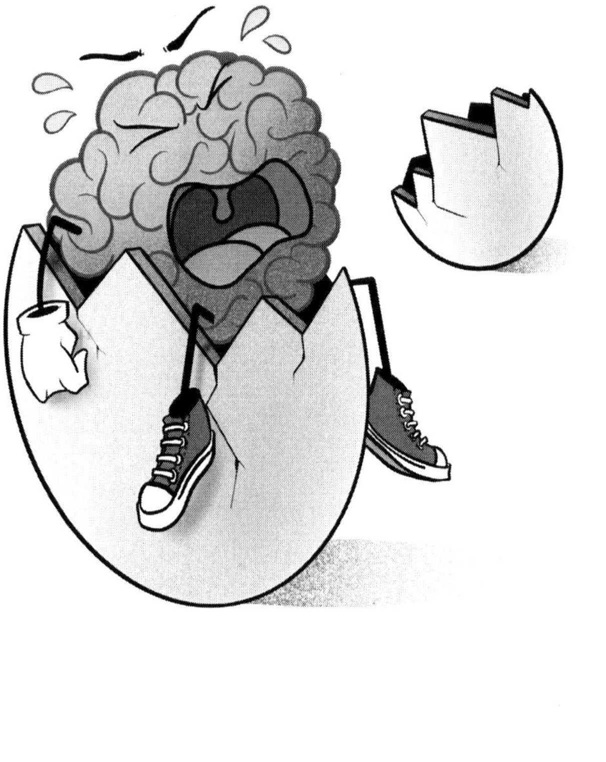

INTRODUCTION

This is not a book of poems or a fairy tale. Some parts will come close to science fiction. There will be drama, myth, and fantasy. I'll try to use humor to give you some insights about what goes on behind the scenes in dental offices, and I promise only one or two horror stories.

This is an essay on dentistry. My goal is to educate you, the dental patient – and maybe even the dentist. I wouldn't call it a guide; I've been a reputable dentist for thirty-five years, but still, the insecure part of me rebels against calling it a guide.

By raising your level of knowledge in the dental arena, I believe I can help you make your own decisions concerning your dental care in the same way I've been making decisions for my patients for many years. And there's a bonus: You'll get cues and tips I never gave my patients, because they were my patients and I was their dentist.

Since you don’t know me yet, this might be a good time to tell you where I'm coming from. Later in the book, you'll learn about my accomplishments in the dental field, but I think it's wise to give you some insights into my dysfunctional upbringing and some of its consequences.

Our family comprised five members: my parents, my two siblings, and me. From the time I was twelve years old, we moved from country to country and from city to city, a total of seven times. I felt no sense of belonging. You'd think that if I didn't find it outside, maybe I'd find it within my family, but we weren't that type.

I've spent my life as an outsider, breaking the rules and talking about things that were usually left unspoken, both inside and outside my profession. I had no fear of consequences because I always spoke the truth – my truth – and always presented it in a well-documented package. Whatever the topic, no matter who were the experts and who had published what, once I acquired enough personal experience and knowledge, I went public with my conclusions if any of those any preestablished dogmas lacked integrity and truth, and believe me, there is an array of them. I became an outspoken, out-of-the-box storyteller. No one could pay me to lie.

No doubt you reckon I didn't find a sense of belonging among my colleagues either – and believe me, this book also won't help matters. The only place I did find my tribe was in my office, among my patients. This wasn't transference; it was my reality.

My patients have given me an only chance to be who I am. No masks, no shame, no fear. I hope this book will show you how important *you* can become to a medical professional regarding your treatment, and why some of those in the field behave differently from the rest of the herd. If you choose the right person, you can have a productive, two-way relationship, which will go a long way toward receiving the proper treatment.

For me, dentistry wasn't about the money or the glory. It was way bigger. It was how I survived, and it made me thrive. Every day, I tried to repay patients for what they were unknowingly giving me. I became the best professional I could be.

My Goal for this book is:

- To clarify any dental problems you may have, without going into too many technicalities, but enough that you can use this book as a reference. It will not be about a specific filling, root canal, , or crown. Instead, we will discuss what goes through your mind before, during, and after any of those procedures, choosing and making sense of it all.
- To explain the emotional piece in dental

treatments and how it affects you and the dental team.

- To analyze the current state of the dental profession and what it can offer in this new millennium.
- To analyze the current state of the dentist, you might be considering, and what he or she has to offer based on age and training. There can be considerable differences between seemingly "similar" dentists.
- To help you become the *real* decision-maker in your treatment plan.

Consider the following:

Even if you choose to be a passive patient and "get out of the way" so that the necessary work can be carried out with the best possible outcome, you will still need to make decisions both at the beginning and as you move forward. As you will discover in this book, your choices can be life-changing.

On what will you base your choice of dentist: On a friend's or your mother-in-law's recommendation? On how charming the dentist is? (That's a dangerous one, not that the mother-in-law one isn't.) On the location of the dental office? (Really?) Will you feel reassured by a few reviews on Yelp, as if your dental treatment is the same as an Amazon purchase, or by a couple of YouTube videos on how a procedure is done? Hmm….

Just to be clear: We're not talking here about a filling or a dental cleaning. We're talking about the oral rehabilitation that you've needed for so long; something which has been affecting your life regarding how you interact with others and how you chew your food. It will often cost you a lot more than an arm and a leg – a kidney and two ribs? – but you can still live without them. In light of this, how long do you usually spend with the dentist before making what can be the decision of your life: forty-five minutes to an hour?

You need more than a chat with a random dentist, more than Yelp; you need the tools to make a proper decision, the right decision *for you.* We will discuss treatments, costs, and expectations – yours, not the dentists. I will show you how important defining your needs and expectations is, and how accepting that you might have to change them and give up control can improve the long-term success of your dental treatment.

Our life is often driven by limiting beliefs about various issues and informed by our personal story, and our attitude toward dental health is no exception. Throughout my life, when I would speak to patients from two distant regions within the same country, I would often get mixed reactions and different requests. Our overall education, our socioeconomic origin, and the conversations our parents had during dinner when we were kids affect our choices when it comes to selecting one dental option over another, or even choosing between two dentists. Here's an example.

I had been practicing dentistry for fifteen years. A woman came into my office. She was around thirty-five, and as pretty as she was austere. All she said was, "I want you to solve the problems in my mouth. I don't care about the cost. I had a car accident six months ago. My eight-year-old son died. I hit my face against the steering wheel. ¨

I was appalled. It was possibly the lengthiest conversation she and I had during almost two years of dental treatment. In light of what she went through, I understood she wanted to be as passive as she could be and needed me to take full control of her dental plan of action. She neither wanted to talk nor had the willpower to make decisions. But what exactly did she want? I had to figure it out and do the best I could with the means I had. For well over eighteen months, until we finished and she moved to Paris, I cared for her as if she had been my child – because she was. I was overwhelmed by the level of trust she had laid at my feet.

Our patients are our children. When you go to the dentist, you become, more than ever, the child, a helpless creature, with an added challenge most of the time – fear.

This is the only way I found to care for patients; therefore, it was my approach to writing this book.

Chapter 1
A Bit of Personal Background

I was born…lol, no. [Joke.]

Thirty-five years of anything is too much. I was a dentist for approximately 12,775 days. I practiced at the highest professional level. I was a surgeon, a teacher, and a lecturer. I poured all the insecurities I had accumulated in my childhood into becoming the best at what I did. For as long as I owned a private practice in Europe, and then Africa, my appointment book was never empty. I always had more work than I could handle.

In what was my success rooted?

- Personal history. Because of the many struggles I experienced during my childhood when I graduated from dental school, I did not think I would make a good dentist. As a young girl, every time my mother came upon me holding a breakable object, I would look at her or just feel her presence, and in a fraction of a second, my grip would loosen. With the help of my good friend gravity, whatever I was holding would shatter. Her preferred commentary was, "Love, become a ballet dancer, not a dentist."

My mother's conviction that I could not be gentle with fragile objects incentivized me to focus on developing techniques to be soft and avoid causing pain. To me, that was the most important thing. If I didn't hurt patients, it wouldn't matter whether I gave the right treatment or not (since I clearly wasn't gifted); patients would simply love coming to me. It worked.

I excelled in ways of placing my hands with the lightness of a feather, and my technique became as gentle as silk. To the very last day I practiced dentistry, patients told me I had the best hands they had ever felt. I read every book I could find on dental anesthesia to perfect my technique, and the needle became my best friend.

- Technique. During my first year out of dental school, the owner of the dental lab I worked with called me one day and asked me to come over. He gave me a tour of the facilities and introduced me to the staff. He then took me into a quiet area and showed me some models made from impressions I had taken. He told me politely and gently that I didn't know what I was doing, and that the (lack of) quality of my work was perforce causing theirs to be substandard. He offered to help me. Strike One in the ego department.

This was the first time I used criticism to up my professional game. I took it well, thanking him for both having the willingness and spending the time to train me.

Later, when I introduce the members of the dental team, you will understand how uncommon it is for a doctor to listen to a lab technician – and even more so to become his student.

From that moment on, realizing how little I knew (close to nothing, although I couldn't tell anyone), I decided to work only with the best. I knew the best would be the most demanding, and it would enable me to climb to the top of my game. It worked.

- Training. Concerning my degree – and please, professors, forgive me if this hurts – I don't believe it is important to know what university a dentist comes from. The differences between training exist, but there is no guarantee of getting a better professional even if you tap into the best university around. Americans might prefer an American-trained dentist, and perhaps Spaniards will also prefer American trained doctors due to a higher country-related reputation. Dental schools, within the same country, vary in quality. But some countries do transmit a better overall dental culture and ethics – which adds up to better care. Summarizing, dental quality can be more country related than university-related. Now, let's look at what happens at the postgraduate level.

Some dentists spend their lives accumulating CE credits[1] through conferences and professional magazine subscriptions or by watching webinars. Seriously? That doesn't work because it's not enough! We are discussing here a highly technical, rapidly evolving, hands-on profession. Would you hire a football player based on how many sports magazines he reads? Yaha. Same. Don't hire dentists who value their comfort zone more than doing real hands-on programs yearly, or who don't have one or several specialized postgraduate credentials. Dentistry is a profession that implies a high level of

[1] CE (continuing education) credits are required in certain countries to maintain our dental licenses. Europe is not so much into CE credits, but the United States is. A magazine subscription will give CE credits, as will attending conferences or symposia, and watching – or should I say playing – a webinar. One can get CE credits for attending private courses as well. In my humble opinion, requiring continuing education for dentists is essential, but not enough.

almost full-time devotion. A dentist who is not committed to learning is committed only to earning. If you have a doubt, get out.

Does this mean you should request a dentist's résumé before you hire him or her? Because that *is* what you're doing; you're hiring them. You should not even have to ask for it. If you check a dental office's website and don't see any résumés, this is a subliminal affirmation that your business is more important to them than their training. Granted, they may have forgotten to upload them onto the website, so go ahead and request to see them.

So yes, my success was also based on my training. As I grew into being a dentist, dentistry grew on me. I knew what I was doing, and when I felt I didn't, I looked for the best and got the training. There is no other way. It worked.

- Grit versus talent. Hands down, grit wins. I am not saying there aren't any excellent naturally gifted dentists out there. But having lived and worked in a country where manual talent is epigenetically transmitted and unquestioned, talent alone, without brain and the grit to study, read and learn are a time bomb. I also see how the most gifted classmates turned out (badly). Look for the hardworking professional; it's safer.

Grit combines courage – taking calculated risks when others won't; conscientiousness; perseverance; resilience; and passion. Excellent dentists need them all. They don't need looks, a pleasant demeanor, a great hairstyle, charm, or a sense of humor – which I also have – unless you plan to marry one. I'm not saying that if you run into a gorgeous, blue-eyed, tall, and athletic dentist you must get up, say you are double-parked and leave, never to come back. Just remember that it's a dentist you're hiring, so don't behave like an untethered adolescent.

➢ Gratitude. Gratitude is the essence of patient care. Foremost, being grateful for having been chosen by you, the patient. It also entails:

- An awareness of the financial effort required to pay our fees.
- An awareness of the physical effort required to reach our office. In some cities, it may take the patient over an hour to reach our location and then maybe an extra hour to park!
- An awareness of where you're at from a dental perspective, and – most important – how you got there. Are you in a dental mess because of

fear? Because of previous financial impediments? Because of a recent accident?

Every time a patient walked into our office, I was full of gratitude, and I would show it. We cherished our patients and pampered them to make sure they would remember how they felt emotionally rather than what they felt physically. I loved greeting them and fetching them from the waiting room when I could, because it made them feel as unique as I felt being their doctor.

Chapter 2

The Team

The concept of dental clinics is becoming more popular throughout the world. Creating a dental office requires a minimum investment of $300,000, usually a lot more. Because dentists, in general, lack the business training related to how setting up and managing a dental practice, big groups (often but not always connected to insurance companies) have come into the picture with visions of the big bucks on the bottom line.

This can be a positive model because it gives business professionals the power to deal with logistics, human resources, equipment, and marketing while allowing the dentists to focus solely on their profession. The situation becomes tricky; however, if the dentists in a group practice do not have full clinical decision autonomy and are bound to unrealistic productivity goals.

If your prospective dentist's office belongs to a group (called a DSO in the United States), how can you find out whether he or she will have the authority to make treatment decisions based only on your needs? First off, do your research with due diligence. This may or may not involve a direct conversation with the practitioner, as groups, being financially oriented, generally prefer to market their brand rather than a specific professional. Which would *you* prefer: knowing the skill you need for correct treatment is in the hands and ethics of an expert or a brand? Some DSOs will preserve the individuality of their doctors and specialists, and in that case, you have nothing to worry about.

The *team* that comprises a dental practice is made of beautiful human beings who dedicate their lives to a fascinating health profession, but with markedly distinct levels of training and often disparate backgrounds.

The dentist is surrounded by dental hygienists, dental assistants (which are called dental nurses in some countries), a front desk team, and often a practice manager. Also, depending on the country, there can be specialties within the profession. When this is the case, coordination and communication among the dental team must be appropriately handled.

Sometimes, but not always, a dental laboratory, staffed by lab technicians ("lab techs"), shares space with the office. This can be a different business entity with separate management or not. Whichever the case, consider it a part of the dental team. Alas, it is not always the case.

If I try to go in-depth into the psychological aspects of the interactions within the dental team, this will no longer be the essay I intend it to be but will resemble an epic science fiction, four-hundred-page manuscript. Not to mention that they'll ban me from most dental clinics around the world and I'll be reduced to performing self-cleanings and self-fillings from now on (which might happen anyway).

Just as I believe dentistry is among the most challenging occupations there are, the dentist is possibly one of the most neurotic professionals there is. Remember: I'm a dentist, so bear with me.

There are two reasons that dentists have a 99 percent divorce rate and a 70 percent rate of suicidal thoughts (we rank first in actual suicides as well). One is what I call the "willpower pump," and the other is the direct effect of rewiring our brain. The willpower pump is a process that takes place every day, almost routinely. While you are sleeping at night, your willpower reservoir gets replenished, and you start the new day fresh, full of will perform a whole slew of tasks and face thousands of challenges. As the day progresses, things don't always go your way, and you must push that massive rock of obligation up your emotional Kilimanjaro. Your stock of willpower gets depleted, and you can accomplish less and less.

As dentists, as we must adapt to eight or ten patients a

day, our willpower also diminishes. The more significant the emotional gap between the patient and us, the more energy is required to breach it. We have to adapt to every patient that enters our office and connect at a deep level, despite the differences in education, cultural baggage or social origin. The more patients we see, the bigger the effort. Our resilience gives in.

As for rewiring our brains, the concept is interesting to say the least.

Imagine that every day as you wake up, I give you a box with tennis balls combined with golf balls, and I ask you to separate them and place them in two different containers. We do this ten times a day for a year.

One evening, you go to a friend's house for dinner. He plays tennis and golf. When you arrive, you see a vase next to the couch with a few tennis balls and some golf balls mixed inside. What will you want to do?

Whether you go ahead and do it doesn't matter. Your eyes will be "REMing" back and forth to the vase throughout the evening. You want to get up and organize it like a crooked painting on the wall, right? It might even unconsciously alter your mood during the evening, so you take the vase and stick it behind the curtains. If your friend is a dentist, you're okay. If not, who knows?

Now imagine that for the next five, ten, fifteen years, we do the same thing with grains of salt and pepper. Can you imagine what would happen if you're in a restaurant and you see a grain of pepper in the saltshaker? Can you imagine how anxious this would make you, since every day, time after time, you separate the black grains from the white? What you are feeling right now is what we call a neurotic behavior.

The dentist works on tiny surfaces eight to ten hours a day. Often a millimeter can alter the outcome of a treatment. Add to that the noise permeating the treatment room and the fact that if you get scared, you might grab my hand anytime, jump, or scream. What will be my stress level when you leave the dental chair? How do you think I will react if there is a fly in the room?

If you are the second most annoying patient in the office that day and two hours before seeing you I treated the first most annoying one, how do you think my neurotic connections and my willpower will handle you? Come on, think! You're already making me nervous, see? No, I cannot explode and throw your denture out the window (first thing that comes to my mind), so to control my reactions with you, explosions will be rerouted to the team, and then to my loved ones at home.

Yes, there are rules, like not scheduling two red-listed, annoying patients on the same day (pro tip).

Dental assistants and, to a lesser extent, hygienists, have the most challenging position in the team. Unless the management has the right level of awareness, we often undervalue their work – and pay them according to our misguided perspective. Undervaluing dental assistants is more often linked to their training and experience than to their responsibilities and the pressure they endure, which is very unfair. I have always been a fervent defender of dental assistants.

As for the lab techs, there is nothing much to say. They are consistently wrong. It is continuously their fault because first, we are neurotic, and second, we have six-plus years of undergraduate training plus often as much in postgraduate credentials, and they don't. So they cannot be right or know more than we, even in their profession. Uh, right?

In fact, their specialty is undergoing lightning changes as technology has rapidly caught up with the dental profession. Most dental work is now digitally milled by machines or printed with 3D printers. The "craftsman" side of dental technology has been highly minimized, requiring fewer lab techs, but with different skills.

I take my hat off to a branch of our industry that has

always had a tough time dealing with us dentists, with our usual arrogance and lack of empathy toward them. The dental lab is the one that makes your dentures, veneers, crowns, onlays, and bridges. (Please refer to the Glossary of Treatments for more information about these vital appliances.) Behind every prosthetic[1] device we deliver, there is always, in the background, a fantastic dental technician or team.

At this point, you can understand how, with this level of disparate teams and skills in addition to psychological disharmony, undeniable communication gaps occur in the field of clinical dentistry. As they cannot always be bridged, they will trigger unspoken errors – what some might consider collateral damage

---

[1] A prosthetic device or dental prosthesis is made by a dental lab and placed in your mouth by a dentist. Its role to rebuild partially destroyed teeth or to replace missing teeth to restore oral function, aesthetics and health.

Chapter 3

Your Dental Problems: A Path to empathy

Have you noticed how close the word *dental* is to *mental*? Just saying.

If there is a branch of healthcare that holds a tighter connection with the psyche than dentistry, I have yet to hear of it. With this statement, I am no longer targeting the dentist. I am talking about you, the patient.

The psychological consequences of childhood or long-standing tooth issues on patients are tremendous. A girl who fractures her central incisor (i.e., her front tooth) at the age of ten can have trauma for life. Front teeth can also go as far as representing masculinity for men.

The first thing a kind and empathetic dentist must do is listen. We will need to understand your language and assess your "dental trauma level." So please, talk openly. Leave your shame at home or in the car. This is essential when it comes to aesthetics because it is the most subjective aspect of dentistry – well, pain is too, but we will discuss that later. Your upbringing, your socio-cultural background, and again, those damn limiting beliefs determine your self-perception. If you don't express yourself unabashedly, we cannot fully understand all aspects of your request, and we will fail *together*.

Then comes our advice. Sometimes, patients ask for things we know will not look good, and it is up to us to guide you, and perhaps help you lower your expectations to get a long-lasting result.

At the beginning of this book, I said this volume is not a guide, and it isn't. But *we* are.

Not all dentists will have the innate aesthetic eye of Leonardo (da Vinci, not DiCaprio), but they may still be able to give you the appropriate treatment. Da Vinci established some golden rules of facial aesthetics, and we abide by them, with or without the gift. Many dentists who do not have this innate talent can develop it with experience. Remember: grit vs. talent.

Dentists must see almost immediately what is wrong in a smile. We need not tell you directly or tactlessly, but we ourselves must know what the problem is. Next, you lead us with your words, and often emotions, through the journey that got you there, and you tell us where you want to go. We must carefully follow and pick up on every verbal nuance and bit of body language as you express your needs, wishes, fears, and frustrations. Sometimes you cry, and that's okay. Often, we can get a picture of your personality and your expectations in less than thirty minutes. We develop that talent, and then it becomes a gift.

Psychology is one of the most fascinating aspects of the dental profession. In order to properly diagnose our patients, dentists must possess, figuratively, 5G antennas to pick up patients' subtle emotional frequencies. Choose a professional who has empathy and who *listens*. Look for cues. A tuned-in dentist must ask the right questions, perhaps to lead you further in your story or to make you see details you are omitting subconsciously or not.

You might be the CEO of a multimillion-dollar company and drive a Tesla, but you're looking for the same thing I am: love and compassion. Yes, even in a relationship with your dentist. Some of you might throw this book out the window right now; why not give it to your partner or other loved one, saying, "Honey! I have a book you'll love!" If one of you reads it, it will serve its purpose.

Good dentists need a well-furnished brain and the use of their analytical mind for many aspects of the profession. But to be a good practitioner in any medical specialty, we need empathy and compassion first. You'll probably be able to pick up on this at your first appointment, but if you're not sure, ask for a second appointment and discuss things further. If you still don't know, try another dentist, no matter what you have heard about the first one.

Sometimes dental treatments can take two years. You will go through moments of doubt, pain, and sometimes despair and rage. You need someone who will understand and empathize. Fifty percent of the dental treatment equation – and thus its success – is the patient, no matter who the doctor is.

There is a second group of professionals who have their own perspective on this: the rest of the dental team.

There is a considerable challenge in treating dental patients under local anesthesia, as one has to deal with "live" anxiety in the form of an ambulatory dental patient. It creates stress on the team, and the patient's reaction will often determine how things go. If you are aware of your stress, your fears, your trauma (most people are), acknowledge them. By suppressing any of them because of appearances and your "need to be strong" – oh, my, that sentiment – you will fuel those emotions and make them more powerful. No one can win that battle. You are vulnerable, and so are we; yes, so are we. Embrace your vulnerability – or read Brené Brown. When my patients do this, I immediately feel good. I know one demon, fear, is under control. We can sense the connectedness between you, me, and the other team members. We're good.

If you're in for a six-, twelve-, or twenty-four-month treatment, disconnection is not suitable. It's just like living detached from your own family, because that is what we become.

For connection to happen, you must acknowledge your fears, but also let go of control. Surrender to the outcome by trusting the team you have chosen. You're on a plane, and you're not the pilot. So let go, and stop going into the cockpit every five minutes to check what they're doing or how you can help.

Fear can turn into phobia, its extreme manifestation, and yet, we still need to treat you. More times than I can remember, I've told patients to take a Valium. If they refused, I would offer to take one myself, so that at least one of us could relax. That would allow them to let go.

As dentists, we are almost by definition empathetic. But how much empathy are you, as the patient, able to develop toward the dental team? Aha! You thought this essay would help you unleash your hatred toward one or two dentists, and that's it? Indeed not. Summon your vulnerability, and let's go through this like the sensible human beings we are, *together*.

As I mentioned, you are hiring a dentist – and the entire dental team – to do the work. Dental treatment is not your Tesla. You don't have to drive it. The driver – the dentist – is a skilled person who needs to be on top of everything and perform a technical task consistent with the current state of the art. No computer tells us what to do or how to do it.

no doubt, your work will come out as close to perfect as humanly possible, but please remember that there's no autopilot…"

Don't think it's any different because you're paying a low, medium, or high fee. Stop thinking that going to the most expensive will be a warranty against defects in craftsmanship. You're not buying a giant TV screen. The quality of the person wearing the scrubs is not in direct proportion with the fee he or she is charging you.

What got you here won't get you there. Trust the journey, make the efforts, and give up your mental resistance to pursue the dental path to your oral health.

Chapter 4
Grinding and Clenching

Now this is important, so listen well. I mean, really listen. Focus on what you read as you repeat in your mind every sentence in this chapter. The subject is important enough for me to devote an entire chapter to it. What you will read can save your natural teeth, your investment, and your mental well-being, and you will soon see why. There's a reason why we're discussing this before any other technical details.

The person who has taught me the most on this topic is Dr. Gene McCoy of San Francisco, one of my three mentors and a close friend. He has dedicated his life to discovering and understanding how, through grinding (also called the Dental Compression Syndrome), patients destroy both their teeth and the restorations we dentists have made for them.

The dental profession has acknowledged Dr. McCoy's research and conclusions, but not in proportion to their implications. There wasn't enough money in it for anyone…except for you, the patient. How? By protecting your ten- or twenty-thousand-dollar oral restoration investment with simple procedures or a night guard that will cost you around $200. Dr. McCoy is the only one who was concerned about safeguarding, if possible, your natural dentition (preventing your existing teeth from mechanical stress breakdown), and if not, at least your dental work. But that's how dentistry and most medical specialties work. If there isn't a big pharmaceutical lab behind it or a specialty within the profession, making millions, you won't know something even exists. Silence kills.

- On occlusion:

Occlusion is how your teeth touch when you close your mouth. Based on the anatomy of your teeth, contacts between teeth can be as subtle as a ballet dancer's feet or as destructive as an elephant's foot. Whether we're talking about your teeth or our restorations, it's the same. Your teeth may have been worn down through years of grinding. If so, you may have transformed what were subtle contacts into massive surfaces rubbing against each other. The forces applied on your teeth will be quite different in either case. Crowns or other restorations may have been made by a lab that doesn't apply the rules we are discussing here, and from day one, your crown has been an elephant foot. This can also happen when a dentist spends an hour-plus adjusting the bite on your new crown with a burr (you know that instrument used to grind down your teeth ?), thus removing the existing cusps[2] and turning the tooth into a paw; one of my teachers used to call it a cooking pan. (Do you know that elephants walk on their toes? Pro tip.)

Above, I mentioned forces. Yes, your mouth is as much a biological organ as a magnificent piece of engineering. It is a biomechanical entity. If we focus on the biology without considering the mechanical aspect, treatment will fail every single time. You will change dentists after they re-cement your crown three times, and you might even swallow it.

It's not in a dentist's best interest to have to repeat a job three times; after all, it takes time, and time is money, but he doesn't know better. Man sees what man knows, and most professionals, too, don't know better. Why? Because the biomechanical implications of our work are generally not taught. We must learn them ourselves. If we're not committed to learning, we're committed only to earning. We must find the right resources wherever they are and choose the best, such as Dr. McCoy. When I heard about his work, I jumped on a plane and went to meet him. Then I invited him to Europe to share his knowledge at our advanced training

[2] Cusps are the four existing pics on the molars, and two on each premolar. Canines also have one cusp.

institute. People listened, but not enough.

- On grinding and clenching:

Grinding, also called bruxism, is not a twentieth- or twenty-first-century problem. It has always been one. Let me cite Dr. McCoy here:

"The flattened teeth in the skulls of our ancestors are dramatic evidence that the untoward condition of clenching and grinding of one's teeth has been in existence since the beginning of time. There are several references to the gnashing of teeth in the Bible (Psalm 35:16, Psalm 112:10, and Job 16:91), but it is an earlier reference that documents the seriousness of the disorder. Clay tablets from the royal library of the Assyrian king Ashurbanipal reveal that grinding of one's teeth was considered both dangerous and pathognomonic as far back as the seventh century BC.[3] *"*

The forces applied on teeth when we sleep are amplified, first because we are asleep, and second because they are sheer lateral forces. Also, we do it all night. It is an endless cycle; all night, every night.

Clenching is a bit less dramatic because we're not ice skating with our teeth, we're holding them tightly

---

[3] Gene Mc Coy, DDS - Look at an old disease. Dental compression syndrome- Journal of Oral Implantology - Vol. XXV/No. One/1999

together, just like John Wayne did to look more manly. It's also something we do both day and night endlessly. What are the conclusions of all this, aside from the fact that most of us are dysfunctionally stressed and should be seeing a psychiatrist?

You are possibly grinding or clenching if:

- You wake up with jaw pain or tightness.
- You have frequent headaches.
- Your teeth have unexplained, general sensitivity to cold, and maybe to hot.
- You keep breaking fillings or restorations, or you are chipping teeth.

Small aside about chipping teeth: Don't think you are original when you say you chipped a tooth biting on this or that. The issue is not *how* you chipped the tooth. Listen to the dentist and let the dentist explain: yes, you might know *when* you chipped it, but not *how*. What made the tooth thin enough to break is the endless cycle of grinding. It follows the same principle as fracturing a paper clip by bending it repetitively. It is called mechanical fatigue. Aren't we subtle with our neurotic behavior?

Bruxism or clenching can also cause:

- Bone loss, or gum recession. By the way, the more you stick your nail where the recession is to check how it is doing today, the more you cause your gums to recede with your germs.

- Grooves at the neck of the teeth (the area closest to the gum). And guess what? They're called McCoy's Notches. Many dentists will tell you they are caused by brushing too hard. You can teach them something new.
- A wavy appearance on the surface of the tooth, more often noticeable on the two front incisors.

What to do? See a dentist and request a night guard. If the first one says you don't need it, see another dentist!

You may also require selective grinding to restore proper soft contacts on your teeth. Not that many practitioners will offer it, but you might get lucky.

Very few dentists will know why you have those notches or waves, so you might want to tell them. At this stage, you possibly already know more about the consequences of bruxism than 80 percent of dentists, no joke.

There are a few qualified, well-trained, and conscientious colleagues, but you might have to do some legwork to find one. Your dentist should offer you a nightguard once he or she has finished your prosthetic work, but if you are not offered one, ask for it. If you have a nightguard made, at the very least, it will stop you from breaking natural teeth, fillings, or any restoration. There are different types of appliances. Please refer to the Glossary of Treatments for more information. By the way, if you wear a denture, you don't need a nightguard; all you must do is remove the denture at night.

Chapter 5

Aesthetic Challenges: Color, Shape, and Position

Let's start with aesthetic challenges with regard to healthy teeth. If you are in this category, you will fit into one of the following two scenarios:

- Although you have a healthy mouth overall, you've hated your smile since childhood because of your teeth's position, shape, or (dis)color. The time has come to grab your teeth by the roots and do something about it.
- What seemed to be a beautiful smile at the age of twenty is not so much at forty-five. You've had no longtime trauma about this; you just want to look and feel better.

Let me just state that your mental condition is not necessarily proportional to your dental issue. Why? Well, aesthetics is subjective, and we don't all react the same to situations such as off-white teeth or a pimple on the nose. The insecurities engendered by how you feel about your appearance can and will make your mind run wild. You can think that because you are otherwise so charming and have such a great sense of humor, it doesn't matter if you have a crooked tooth. But you might instead believe that the reason you got fired, are getting divorced, and missed your flight is because of your dental issues. (Actually, you might miss a flight if you take too long to floss your crooked teeth.)

Let's use a bit of Cartesian reasoning and separate the aesthetic dilemma into three components: Color, shape, and position.

1. The color of your teeth

If you are disturbed by the color of your teeth, there are several questions a dentist must ask you:

Are they yellow? Like, too yellow, but the rest –shape and position – is perfect?

Do you brush your teeth? I mean, *really* brush your teeth. You can't imagine what we see in dental offices – including worms under a denture that a patient hasn't taken out in five years – so just bear with me and with what you might consider silly questions.

Let us assume you brush your teeth, and you use a toothbrush you have bought within the past three months. Let us also assume you go for checkups and cleanings every six months but not less than once a year. You've also tried, along with the brushing and the cleaning, any system of dental air abrasion such as AquaCare®, Prophy-Jet®, or another similar product, which removes superficial stains. If after all this, your teeth are still yellow, then you have a number of options. Plan A: Think about the last time you had an argument with someone. Did you start calmly, segue into assertive, and then eventually become aggressive? Likewise with dealing with discolored teeth, you go from conservative to more aggressive. Get a teeth **Whitening** done before going any further. (Not in the middle of an argument with a loved one, smart aleck.)

Whitening is the first step. Contrary to popular belief, having your teeth whitened by a professional does not damage them. What we do in a dental office is not comparable to anything you can buy over the counter and off the shelf. We use concentrations and specialized products that are much more efficient. We also use ultraviolet light or laser to activate the product, which enhances its whitening potential. If you want full-on efficiency, a professional whitening always has to be followed by at-home bleaching with custom-made bleaching trays for at least two weeks. The reason for this is that the slight reversible alteration of the enamel caused by the product we use in the office will remain for about fifteen days. Therefore, not only can you enhance the result by using a whitening product for as long as the enamel "pores" remain open – it's a metaphor, but close to reality – you can also avoid immediate staining when the enamel is the most prone to it.

It is also of utmost importance during these fifteen days to avoid drinking colored carbonated sodas – which you should avoid anyway at all times, since they also lower your saliva's Ph[4]. Stay away from any foods made with strong coloring agents, such as saffron, turmeric, and even cinnamon. No oranges or their juice, tea, or coffee, red wine, or any other colored drinks. If you have an addiction to any of these, and do not want to desist from consuming it, brush your teeth right after drinking. And Do Not Smoke!

Plan B: If your teeth are very yellow and are resistant to whitening, it may be due to a defect, based on an abnormal buildup of yellower tissue – a category of dentin [5]– below the enamel.

In this case, the next step is doing **Veneers**, also called **Laminates**. This option will also apply to teeth

---

[4] Low saliva's Ph (acid) will increase the risk of cavities

[5] Dentin is the tissue (material) located two millimeters below the enamel of a tooth. There are different categories of dentin. They vary in structure and color. Enamel being semi-translucent, dentin will contribute to the color of a tooth.

discoloration caused by antibiotics–tetracycline -, or any other agent taken during amelogenesis, which is not a rock band but the time during childhood when the enamel is formed. Likewise, some specific regions in Africa, for example northern Tanzania, have problems related to water quality. Thus a significant percentage of the population there have teeth with deep stains that can be corrected only with veneers.

A veneer is a thin laminate generally made of porcelain (which gets more beautiful results than other materials), which is placed on the surface of an anterior (front) tooth to correct a defect in color or shape or mild defect in position. The dental lab makes it; therefore, it requires at least two appointments.

An amount of enamel equal to the thickness of the veneer will have to be removed from your tooth to respect the biological environment of the restoration. While the veneer is being made, you will have to wear a temporary appliance, which can sometimes be as temporary as the amount of time it takes to reach your car. Oh well, as Buddhists say, all is impermanent.

In the right hands, veneers are one of the most successful restorative treatments, and much less invasive than crowns. Although you may end up needing a root canal later because of the anatomy or the position of the tooth, the chances of this happening are less than with a crown. Also, even if you do end up needing a root canal, the risk of future fracture of the tooth is less because overall, veneers remove less substance than do crowns. (By the way, please note that crowns are no-no's if the problem is discoloration, shape, or small defects in position.)

2. The shape of your teeth – and gums

Some necessary information: The shape and harmony of your six to eight anterior teeth are vital to a beautiful smile. But the balance between them and the position of your lips and gums is as important. If the gum line, for example, is at a different level on each front tooth, you might think there is something wrong with the shape of your teeth, but it only takes altering the gum line slightly to bring equilibrium back. This is just one example of many.

If you want to be a good judge of your smile overall, look at a photograph of you with a natural smile on a computer screen. If you look in a mirror, your limiting beliefs will alter what you see. You will notice what your mind wants you to see. In a photograph, you see yourself *as you are*, and your assessment will be less biased. But is judgment ever fair? We'll leave the answer to that for another book.

The question we must always conquer, no matter the patient's goal, is what caused the problem we're meant to solve. The *why* is the key to the solution.

The shape of your teeth may have been altered by previous fillings, or you could have been hit by a tennis racket. Ouch. Those cases are straightforward, no joking, and the procedure of choice is often veneers if there is enough healthy tooth structure to support them. See the above description or the Glossary of Treatments at the end of this book for more information. In extreme cases, the problem could be caused by crowns and thus require root canals, but give me a sec before I digress again, because I will lose you.

The gum line must have harmony and allow all aspects of the teeth to be seen. Sometimes, in patients who are grinders or whose teeth are in the wrong position, the gum has migrated and covers part of the tooth; or there is a recession, meaning the gum is higher than usual. Please see the illustration below. If we do a veneer, we must also correct the gum. If we remove gum, we call it a **Gingivectomy**. (If we add gum, we call it a gingival graft.)

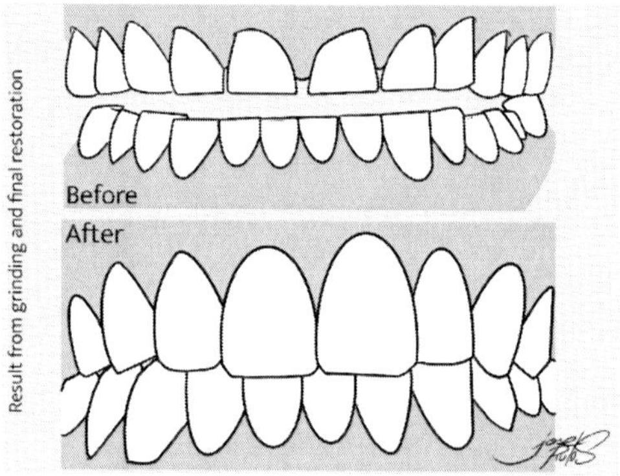

Let me say a word on gum recession and how you, the patient, point them to us by sticking your nail right on it. Do you know how many germs are trapped under your nail? To cite just one bacteria, check out the staphylococcus aureus. Just FYI, it's known to cause, among other things, respiratory infections, food poisoning, skin infections, and abscesses. So what do you think it does to your gum recession or to any other problem you're "pointing out" to us? Stop sticking your fingers in your mouth! You may complain about the edge of your teeth being too thin and grayish-looking because of transparency, or your teeth looking shorter than they did when you got married. This is due to grinding your teeth, which from my experience, 80 to 90 percent of us do. I am not saying that marriage makes you grind, but it could, just as financial or work-related stress can. If you look at your teeth and you don't see the typical vampire canine, or if you see the edges of your teeth being in an almost straight line from canine to canine, you are possibly a grinder. (Not to say that vampires don't grind, or that if you grind you're not a vampire.) So, if it's grinding that has at least partially caused the defect you are trying to correct, and your dentist restores it with veneers or crowns without making you a nightguard, you will break whatever restorations he or she made. Porcelain will break rather sooner than later in the mouth of a grinder. This is the best example of why the "why" is so essential. (In case you skipped it, if you want to know more about grinding, please go back to the previous chapter.)

3. The Position of Your Teeth

You have probably figured out by now that the position of the teeth will always dictate the location of the gum. Thus, when you correct the first, the latter will automatically follow in its wake without other interventions.

In the past year, I have seen at least four young patients request the extraction of beautiful but misaligned canines to get bridges over healthy teeth, thus mutilating six to eight healthy ones and pulling out two – just for the sake of instant gratification. If you agree with these young people, give this book to a friend; it's not for you. In all four cases, I walked into the room and explained to the best of my ability, as a clinical consultant, the error they were making. Had the patients been mine, I would have rejected the treatment as I have always done. We are doctors and should do no harm. **Orthodontics** is the way to go when a canine or any other healthy tooth is in the wrong position.

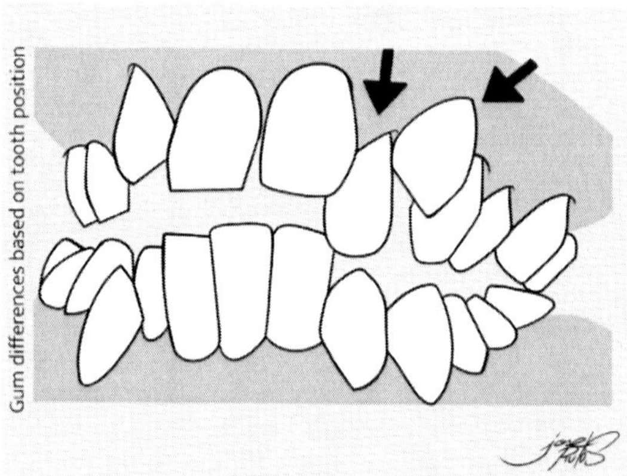

Why do patients refuse the best and least invasive treatment? Generally, it's because of social background, lack of dental education or education overall, and instant gratification. In times where anything can be delivered to your door – sometimes in less than twenty-four hours, you can't expect an uneducated patient to wait twelve to eighteen months to get the desired result.

Why do doctors agree to do it? Instant gratification.
By doing so, we are messing up the dental life of the patient. We would never do it to our daughter, son, or sister. Then why to a patient?
Maybe, just maybe, I could have understood a patient not willing to get braces a few generations ago because of the aesthetic implications. But nowadays, with options such as Invisalign®? These orthodontic treatments use clear acrylic (transparent plastic) guards to restore teeth to their aesthetic and functional positions. They have a level of predictability now often higher than conventional orthodontics, and take less time, too. Please refer to the Glossary of Treatments for details.
Don't get me wrong; sometimes, orthodontics do require the extraction of healthy teeth. But never a canine, and not to speed up a process, but because there is not enough space for very wide teeth in a smaller arch. We call them strategic extractions. In this case, we are often talking about the extraction of premolars[6], not only because aesthetically it is not mutilating once the correction is finished, but also because often premolars

---

[6] We have 8 premolars in total, two in each quadrant, located right after the canines(eye tooth) and before the molars

that end up restored will cause further problems with time.

So the first choice for the correction of teeth position is orthodontics. If we are talking about some slight defects that you cannot live with, a compromise can be one or two veneers for those teeth.

There is something else you need to understand. When a tooth has even a slight misalignment, it will get worse with time. It happens because those teeth are no longer being held in place by the ones next to them. Imagine five soldiers in a straight line pressing against each other at shoulder level with their arms placed against their bodies. If one of them tilts slightly, the pressure from his mates will push him outside the line. The moment one tooth is out of place, even if you correct it with a veneer, it will continue to move unless you splint that tooth. The neighboring teeth don't see the difference; For them, the tooth is out of place, and they continue to exert pressure. Thus, a few years later, the appearance will change again, or the veneer will fall off.

The best way to prevent this scenario is to get a night guard once we make the veneer, just as you would after orthodontic treatment, to keep the teeth in place. It will not only protect your teeth from grinding damage, as we learned above, but it will also stop the teeth from moving by containing them within its boundaries. Wearing it at night is enough. It will undo any movements that happened during your waking hours.

Even if you end up doing nothing at all about the slight misalignment in your front teeth, by getting at least a nightguard, you can feel confident the condition won't worsen because your teeth will stop moving. If you choose not to get a night guard either, then get ready to notice, year after year, how initially slightly crooked teeth become an aesthetic aggravation. You know that Bugs Bunny look? Told ya….

What if your teeth are not healthy? What if, because of dental abandonment based primarily on lousy hygiene and dental laziness, your teeth are a mess? That's a chapter on its own. Follow me.

Chapter 6

When Things Get Messy, The Path to Infection

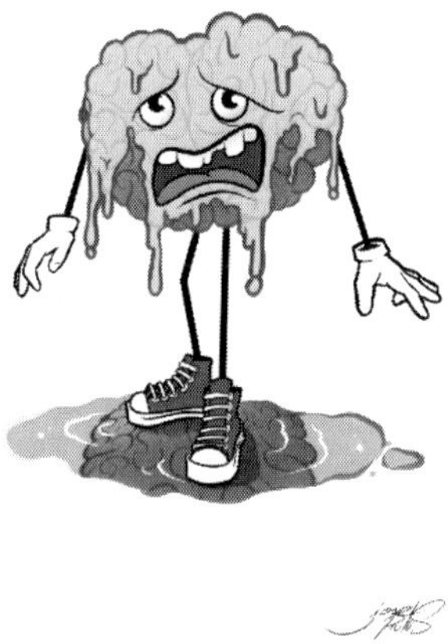

This is it. Let's take a deep dive.

If you are reading this, you may be one of these patients, or you may want to understand what a loved one is going through.

Let me explain the cases we are dealing with here as objectively as I can. Some of you might think I'm not empathetic in this chapter, but thirty-plus years of seeing patients like you and caring as much as I do for your situation and pain has given me some insights.

If I am blunt, it's because I want this book to be a wake-up call. I'm hoping to help many suffering people. I will say things I've never said to any of my many patients, out of fear of causing grief or humiliation, and because once patients were in my office, they didn't need to hear it anymore. All they needed then was empathy and compassion. I have faith that this chapter will be all the incentive you need to get help. Have no fear of being judged by the profession. Self-judgment or judgment from others disappears the moment you act. When you find the courage to step up and face your fear, not allowing it to control your dental outcome anymore, you are on your way.

Your dental story may have started when you were a child, eating candies and drinking sodas, not brushing because you didn't know better. Maybe the caring adults around you didn't know better either. Education, along with dental education, can be linked to the socioeconomic origin or not. Poor hygiene, along with perhaps not-so-good genes and a so-so diet, creates an explosive dental time bomb. Unless at some point, you or a caring adult around you become aware of your oral health, by the age of thirty-five at the latest, you will have a head-on collision with the Tree – a concept I will explain in a few minutes.

It is rare to have a balanced dental education during childhood and find yourself in this mess because you abandoned sound practices, although it can happen. You might have become a substance abuser, at which time oral care became secondary. When you emerged from the tunnel, how many years later, you reap debris in many aspects of your life, and your dental health is no exception. Drugs, especially heroin, alter the quality of saliva, which can then no longer play its role in protecting against bacteria.

Sometimes, a dramatic event in your life or clinical depression takes you to a dark place. Oral care becomes secondary for a prolonged time.

Except for this third scenario, which takes us back to the story I outlined in the Introduction, about the patient who lost her child and destroyed her teeth in a car accident, the journey to declining oral health is consistent. The worse it gets, the less you brush, and the worse it gets. You already didn't go to the dentist much, but now you've decided not to ever go again, because, after all, you are a mess and no one can help you (you said it, I didn't). You victimize and judge yourself. As you do, you believe others will too.

And then, ah, yes! Money! You have no money, so you decide not to care for your teeth anymore and save on visits to the dentist. But you buy cigarettes and booze, and secure a loan to replace the car. Right.

The incredible thing here is that if your six anterior teeth remain intact and allow you to smile, you can remain circling in this same flight pattern. No one will notice. You can even have those anterior teeth repaired if needed, and when the dentist asks you about the rest, you can answer, "Yes, I will do it; give me a quote, please." You take it home and put it with the other three or ten you have. You then continue to place your hand in front of your mouth when you smile, or you pucker up so that others won't see the gaps. But they do.

You alter your facial expressions to cover the defects. You even manage to eat, although half your back teeth are missing!

This discourse will irritate some of you. I could have chosen to be empathetic and compassionate, but the price you will pay is too high. I told you: No one can pay me to lie.

At some point, it becomes a conscious decision to let your oral health reach such a level of wreckage. It is self-destruction. Of course, circumstances haven't helped, but you can change them or make new ones.

Dwelling on the past and playing the victim has led you to where you are.

Einstein said that the definition of insanity is doing the same unproductive thing repeatedly and expecting a different result. It's up to you to handle your poor oral health differently. So step up and take responsibility for it.

For close to thirty-five years, I have treated more than fifteen thousand different patients throughout one hundred thousand appointments. Although no two patients are exactly alike, and conversely, there is no one mold for them all, what makes the clinical experience valuable is the fact that dental patients fit into, say, ten categories overall. Thus, there is a predictability to their – and your –reactions. Knowing this, I will describe the Tree. Not the Tree of Knowledge or the Tree of Life. The Tree you will collide with if you don't wake up.

Most of the cases I will discuss below involve infected teeth. Let us now take a trip to Africa (no safari included).

I have taken part in humanitarian actions in Tanzania, which is part of East Africa for many years. There, 23 million people have no access to oral care and live on less than a dollar a day. Talk about a harsh socioeconomic background! Their situation is so precarious that we base most outreach camps on dental extractions; most of the time, we don't even try to save teeth.

Many Tanzanian tribes believe in witchcraft. People go to a sorcerer for healing and spells, and this almighty healer does not like to attend our camps. Yet, when one of these sorcerers has a compelling enough reason, they will show up. We immediately know they've arrived because the tribe members whisper and point them out, almost laughing at them. Do you want to know when these healers come for extractions? When they have an infected upper molar or upper canine. They have learned that those can kill. And if *they* know, everybody else does too. In Tanzania, human life is not worth much. Tanzanians deal with death daily and don't even find the tears to cry. But they know one thing better than most people in the western world, including most of the people who are reading this book. They know that dental infections kill. And believe me, their bacteria do not differ from ours.

In thirty-five years, I have seen over a dozen deaths caused by oral complications-related brain abscesses and by oral cancer (which we'll discuss later). And I've seen them not in Africa, but in high-end, private European dental practices. Some of the victims were CEOs. Money and education are not the issues here.

Stubbornness, disbelief, and the need to control your dental outcome because you think you know better can kill you. We can sometimes discern arrogance when we explain this to patients. The "not me" look still gives me cold sweats. The higher the socioeconomic level of the patient, the more this arrogance comes forward and creates a clash with the well-intentioned doctor. Ego comes in, and no one wins.

The biggest ego clash I had with a patient for this exact reason led her to leave my office, almost slamming the door. I diagnosed an infection on a tooth she did not want to treat. "How come no one else has told me this? What do you know that they don't?" That was like a punch in the gut. Although I didn't react, no doubt, my body language did. I said I couldn't answer her question but maintained that we couldn't do any other dental work unless we treated that tooth first. Two weeks later, the longtime patient who had referred this woman to me called to tell me her friend had died. She asked me, "Did she have a dental infection? What happened during her appointment? You know, she didn't like you and went to another dentist." I couldn't answer her questions, as professional secrecy is our first commandment. But I was appalled.

Upper teeth infections create their path to the brain; lower, to the lungs. Any or all of them connect to the heart, kidneys, and every organ via the bloodstream. If everyone who died got an autopsy, the number of people who were discovered to have died of tooth infection-related issues would be much higher than those who died of COVID-19 in 2020, and global focus on the prevention of pandemic death would point in the right direction.

Let us now de-dramatize and talk about what happens before you lose a tooth. First, you get a decay, or what is also called a cavity. Or your troubles might begin with a broken filling, or under an existing crown or restoration.

You begin having sensitivity to cold on that tooth, but you ignore it. You progressively experience episodes of acute pain combined with periods of remission, but you ignore it. Eventually the pain gives you sleepless nights, and you take painkillers and self-medicate with antibiotics you had in your medicine cabinet. You're okay. The pain is gone. You continue to ignore it.

Now you occasionally have a bump on the gum, where the tooth is, but it doesn't hurt. You rinse with mouthwash because you're a dentist wannabe. You are so cool. Who needs to spend $300 seeing someone, right?

By now, the tooth could have broken, sometimes to the gum-level, but symptoms are gone. Now that you know the path to dental enlightenment, you just keep doing the same every time you get a toothache. My question is, would you have done the same if it had been your eye? Your hand? Your foot? Why that behavior with teeth, because you have thirty-two of them? Yes. The only universal thing is ignorance.

What has really happened, and what should you have done? When the filling broke, you should have gone to the dentist and have it checked and replaced. Same thing the moment you felt sensitivity, even if there was no previous filling in that tooth. Let's say the cost would have been around $200.

But instead, you continued to ignore the situation. Bacteria kept doing their thing, which was to destroy your tooth. As they progressed closer to the pulp (also called the nerve), you experienced those episodes of pain. That was a warning. Your body was aching and asking you to care for it as much as it cares for you.

As you ignored the signs, bacteria invaded the pulp, and you end up needing a root canal, which is the treatment that implies the disinfection of the nerve and the placement of medication. If you don't get it done, the tooth gets infected. From this point onward, the infection grows, and grows, and grows. Now, treatment can range from $450 to $1,200 depending on what tooth is involved and the dentist you go to. Then, after the root canal, the tooth will have to be rebuilt, often with a post, and probably with a crown. Now you're in for over $2,000.

Here’s the equation: $200 + passive dental attitude (PDA) = $2,000. That makes poor business sense.

You don't have the money or don't want to spend that amount on a tooth you say you'll lose anyway? Ask the dentist to pull it out; at least it's smarter than keeping the infection. This will set you back $110–$200, so you're back where you started from but mutilated. (Because that’s what an extraction is – a mutilation.)

Replacing the extracted tooth, assuming that's possible based on several number of technical criteria, will cost you between $3,500 and $7,000. The price depends on whether you get a three-unit bridge or an implant, and whether the teeth that will support the bridge need further treatment or you need a bone graft to place an implant (those last two scenarios account for the higher estimate). Here, the equation is $200 + PDA= $3,500–$7,000. Once again, prices will also vary from one practitioner to the next. We'll learn more about this in chapter 8.

Foremost takeaway: Don't think you have it under control. If you don't want to or can't be treated because of finances, have the diseased tooth pulled out! Be at least as smart as our underprivileged Tanzanian patients!

Once you lose a tooth to extraction, the cheapest solution for its replacement is a removable appliance. It can be a full denture – all fake teeth – or a partial one, with just a few phony teeth. If you can get a partial denture (meaning that you have some natural teeth left), try to get a metal-based one, as it is better for the remaining teeth, and it will be more comfortable.

If you chose not to replace missing teeth in the back because your front ones are still solid, and you have decided you will not wear a denture, know that you will lose the remaining front teeth quickly. Your mouth is a biomechanical entity where forces can be immense. Often you refuse the partial denture because of limiting beliefs and social stigmas, but you're falling off a twenty-story building, and it will hurt when you hit the ground.

The molars you have lost were there to protect the fragile anterior teeth. If they're not replaced, all forces are transferred to the most anterior ones, destroying them one by one. Following this same principle, if you do crowns or a bridge on anterior teeth because you're all about aesthetics but don't replace the posterior teeth because you don't want to give up your ski holidays, the investment in the front teeth would be the equivalent of buying and driving a Tesla with three wheels. Unfortunately, many dentists will push you to restore at least prosthetically – with crowns and bridgework – your anterior sector, hoping you will get run over by a car before it fails.

If you can afford a fixed solution rather than a removable (fixed is always more expensive) and have lost quite a few teeth, then the answer will be any of the multiple combinations of crowns on top of natural teeth and implants to replace the missing teeth. You will find details on this in the Glossary of Treatments.[7]

Just remember that implants need bone. When you first lost your tooth, you most probably had bone available, but no money. Now that you have money, you might not have enough bone. You can get a loan for money, but there is no loan for bone. Pick your poison.

When you lose a tooth, you lose bone. The more time goes by, without a tooth, the more bone you lose. Bone

---

[7] More information will also be available in my next book, *Stairway to Implants*, due to come out in late 2020.

– tooth + time = Less bone. Moreover, if you wear a removable denture as you wait for the implant-based solution (meaning until you have the money) and do not take it off at night, you will lose more bone by wearing it. Yes, there are also fifty shades of gray in dentistry.

When there is no bone to place implants, you need a bone graft. These can be expensive since they require highly qualified surgeons, and both treatment duration and cost will increase by as much as 50 percent.

If money is the issue, your best bet is always to get a loan; the earlier, the better. A 10–12 percent interest rate is better than a 50 percent increase in the cost of treatment. Be smart, not proud.

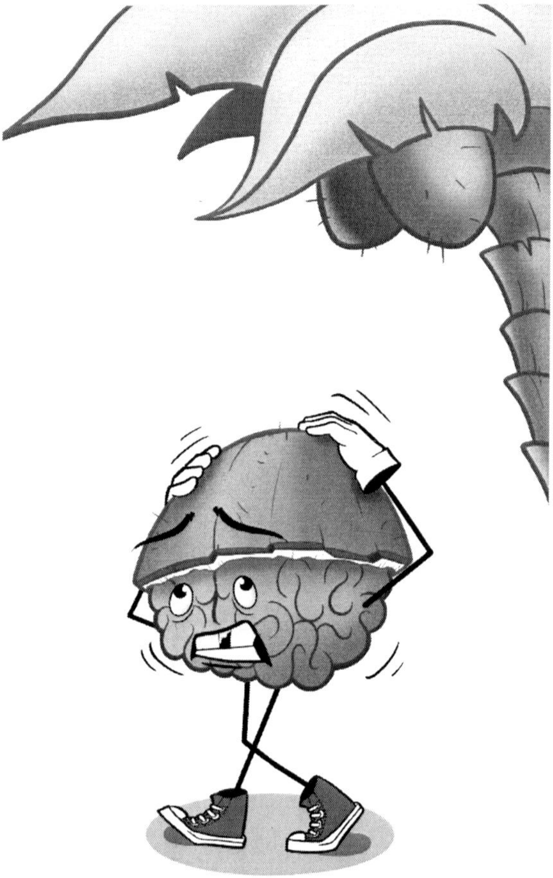

Chapter 7

On Pain, Fear, and the Fear of Pain

I almost feel like putting an ellipsis here and calling it a day. You all have your opinion on this, and you possibly think you know more about pain than I do, right? Wrong.

There is a Lady Gaga song that goes, "Don't be scared, I've done this before. Show me your teeth." Please do not listen to it in the middle of this read, as the song's topic isn't dental…if you know what I mean. Let's just say that fear is free and always readily available.

There is no area of the brain that can be removed to eliminate pain. Fear, on the other hand, is in a small zone called the amygdala. When burned with a needle on rats, they run after cats. Yes.

The origin of pain was to protect the species. Pain is there first to let us know that we are burning, cutting, or otherwise hurting our physical body. Pain and fear will generate a fight-or-flight response through the identification of danger, and that is good. It is the primal life-preservation instinct. But as much as it is valid for all creatures, we humans have a mind, too, and that changes everything.

The Coconut Dilemma

You are standing in front of me, under a coconut tree. We are using you to test my theory on pain. A guy has climbed the tree, and we know he will cut off a branch holding one coconut, which will then fall and hit you on the head. The three of us agreed on this. The theorem we're off to prove is not that a falling coconut can kill you, but that by knowing what will happen in advance, or even better, by *thinking* you know what will happen, you transform what you feel. You imagine the pain. You are pre-immersing yourself in the sensation the coconut will create as it hits your head. This will change the way you perceive the pain when it happens because you are expecting it, so your mind has taken over. Well, because you have never been hit on the head by a coconut before, it is, more precisely, your imagination taking over.

However, if you are standing under a coconut tree without knowing it's a coconut tree, and a coconut falls on your head unexpectedly and luckily does not kill you, since you were not expecting it, your perception of how the impact feels is different. You haven't previously experienced a cognitive process to distort the event. This phenomenon is borne out in situations where people had a limb amputated by a shark, for example, and said they felt no pain. This is how pain works when the recipient did not expect the event that caused it.

There is a second factor in the pain equation, which is whether or not you experienced that exact pain before. Since you have never been hit by a coconut, you don't know exactly how it will feel, so you create an expectation of how you imagine it will feel. Wow. That's a complicated game: We humans are capable of imagining how something we have never experienced will feel, pre-immersing ourselves in the event, and creating the fear associated with it. We base both reactions on two abilities we have: an extremely selective memory and a fertile imagination.

Pain is quite a dragon, and so is fear. They are linked, and the first precedes the latter. They both live in a cave called the mind. People who have not experienced pain at the dentist or heard horror stories during childhood will not fear pain from the dentist.

Now let's see what happens when you go to the dentist.

There are two options: either you are afraid of dentists, or you are not. Nobody likes us, so don't say, "Ugh, I hate dentists!" That's the least original statement I've ever heard.

For animals, fear has one phase. The wildebeest sees the lion – or is it the other way around? – and starts running for its life. It had no fear before it saw the lion, just innate methods to stay safe. If the wildebeest gets away, it will run back to its herd as if nothing had happened, and the event is over. It lives in the now.

As humans, once we've experienced something, or heard about a situation before we've lived it, we pre-immerse ourselves in it, fantasizing and creating all sorts of false emotions. When the event actually happens, we fully immerse ourselves in it, and when it's over, we post-immerse ourselves for days, weeks, months, or even years. Regurgitating fear through our pores is indeed a form of insanity.

Fear of dentists has one of two sources:

- **Your own experience**. You don't have to imagine it. One or many of us have hurt you, and that did it. The connection in your neurons is there until someone disconnects them. Just like the bell and Pavlov's dogs, when you hear the D-word, your blood pressure drops and you get cold sweats. You have a trauma based on your own experience. A coconut has previously fallen on your head.
- **Other people's experiences**. Often, someone will take advantage of family dinnertime togetherness to recount the story of the day's extraction, describing how the dentist placed his knee against their chest and started

pulling with huge pliers. Hearing and almost feeling in your bones how people you loved suffered through dental treatment caused you trauma. Because the subconscious does not distinguish between things you have personally experienced and tales others have told, it is therefore irrelevant whether your emotions are directly connected to an event or created by thought alone; your brain will make the same connections either way. You imagine the scenes, the feelings, and the pain. You are projecting an event into the future.

If you have found or now find yourself at a dentist who causes you unexpected discomfort more than once, I hope you change practitioners. If you’re still seeing the same scary guy or gal, put this book down and immediately get a self-help manual on childhood trauma.

Dental treatment should not hurt. We work under local anesthesia, and when we know what we are doing, it is enough. Every dentist has their own way of placing their hands, using a needle, and doing an extraction. No two dentists are the same, believe me. Techniques can be similar when training is comparable, but not the way we put things into practice.

So if you've had a nasty experience, just change dentists. Don't expect to find the dream dentist on the first try.

Look at everything, not just the fee or how close the office is to where you live. Some people go to a hairdresser an hour away from home and then look for a dentist around the corner. If it's for the kids, it gets even worse; they try to find one in their same building!

Don't assume dental treatment will hurt based on previous experience or horror stories. Give your new dentist a chance, just like you would do with a new friend. Don't compare; start from scratch. All dentists are not the same, just like all men are not the same – or all women, either.

There is a reason dentists have a poor reputation. What can I say? Many entered the profession for the money. To repeat: If they're not committed to learning, they're committed only to earning. No matter how many initials are after your name, if you don't have the drive, the passion, and the vocational influx to be a dentist, you are not a dentist.

But don't despair; there are many exceptionally talented and passionate dentists entirely dedicated to serving patients and deserving your trust. Look for those. Don't settle for less, unless you want to be part of a horror story yourself. Let go of the limiting beliefs you created based on your previous terrible dental experiences (real or imaginary). Remember: you create your own reality.

What others share as their struggle is what they have attracted into their lives based on their fears, their limiting beliefs, and their behavior. If you don't go by what you hear others say about dentists, your search for the right one for you will be "clean"; you'll create a new experience. You will overcome the fear of pain because you know it is nonexistent, both during and after treatment. A dentist who works softly doesn't cause damage to the tissues, and those tissues will, therefore, not suffer. A practitioner who works harshly will cause unnecessary harm, and thus you will experience postoperative pain.

Leave your preconceived ideas and old rags at the door. Give yourself a chance.

Toothaches

Let's discuss toothache here, since it belongs to the category of pain.

If you are in intense pain due to a toothache, I'm sorry to say that it's your fault. I have yet to see a case where a toothache goes from zero to one hundred without a previous warning. It's not sudden like an earthquake. Only if you are in the wrong dental hands and something was done incorrectly can you suddenly be in intense pain from one day to the next, but this is infrequent.

Let's apply the Richter scale to a toothache. Why?

Because it'll be fun, and you'll remember it.

The Richter scale goes from 1 to 10:

- Less than 2: Micro
- 2–2.9: Very Minor
- 3–3.9: Minor
- 4–4.9: Light
- 5–5.9: Moderate
- 6–6.9: Strong
- 7–7.9: Major
- 8–9.9: Great
- 10+: Meteoric (I love this one)

What is the parallel between earthquakes and toothaches? There is none. They work in opposite ways. That's why you'll remember the analogy.

Even a major earthquake can happen without a previous warning. That's why it can cause so much damage and kill so many people. A Richter scale-based toothache, on the other hand, will gradually progress from light to strong to great. If you wait to see a dentist because you think you know better, you'll find yourself with the meteoric pain; pressure-related, intense agony in the middle of the night.

For an 8-point toothache there is no self-medication, because nothing is potent enough. It is one of the most intense pains a human can endure. Why wait? After

thirty-five years, I still don't get it.
I can't wait to see your dentist's face when you say you have a toothache of 6.4 Richter scale-magnitude pain. Hilarious.

Phobias

A phobia is an inexplicable, exaggerated, and illogical fear of an object or situation, as per Merriam-Webster (granted, it's not a psychologist; it's a dictionary).
The most common phobia in our profession is the needle phobia, but I haven't had insurmountable situations with those. I will cut this short by saying that there are better- and worse-quality needles, mostly concerning the design of their bevel. The bevel, which is at the tip of the needle, is what allows us to make the penetration of the needle seamless or unpleasant. Moreover, as you anesthetize multiple areas, the bevel becomes less and less efficient, and the sting more noticeable. A conscientious dentist doesn't worry about spending more for quality needles and using more than one for the same patient. The same happens with Botox injections. Have you noticed how the first two are not all that bad, but by the tenth, you want to rip the doctor's heart out? The right doctor or dentist will be soft enough that you will not even know when he or she is using a needle.
Now, let me tell you a true story that will help you

understand how phobias work.

One day a patient comes to my office, and as I get ready to treat her, she tells me she has a phobia of adrenaline. She explains that she's had this phobia since childhood and that no one has ever been able to treat her with adrenaline because she goes into convulsions and a screaming fit. Hmm.

A few things about adrenaline, also called epinephrine. It is both a medication and a neurotransmitter. As a medication, among other uses, epinephrine is part of the composition of anesthesia. It makes the use of anesthesia safer and restrains bleeding during surgical procedures.

As a neurotransmitter, adrenaline is what your adrenal glands secrete when you go into a fight-or-flight situation; for example, it speeds up your pulse and makes you run when you see a tiger. You cannot survive without it, not just because of the tiger but because you need it. You cannot possibly have an autoimmune attack on adrenaline because your body isn't stupid. Adrenaline contributes to many necessary physiological functions; hence it is needed.

Considering the above explanation, I know that adrenaline can't cause this woman to have convulsions or a screaming attack. I don't tell her this, however.

I was to do minor surgery on the patient, so I anesthetized her with an extremely low dosage of adrenaline-based product. She immediately screamed and went into a crazed reaction. Hmm.

I continue to anesthetize without the adrenaline component, and all goes fine. No response on her end. I am astounded.

As I am finishing up the procedure, she bleeds a bit too much, so to stanch the flow, I inject a few drops of lidocaine mixed with adrenaline into the area. Her eyes are closed, she has taken some sedation because of her nervousness, she is already numb and almost asleep; in other words, she can't feel anything. The instant the product goes in, however, she screams, scares the hell out of me, and goes back into that frantic, cat-like kickback. Jesus, Mary, and Joseph! I thought I would have a heart attack! How can she know? How on earth is that possible, and how can her reaction be so immediate? When I was finished for the day, I shared what happened with a close friend who is a famous psychiatrist specializing in, among other things, phobias. He laughed at me, like ha-ha laughed. He went on to explain that what might have happened was that as a child, when my patient was once injected with adrenaline, her heart sped up because the product went into an artery, which happens sometimes. Though it may be uncomfortable for a few seconds, it's usually not a big deal, but if she was a very fearful type, she might have been terrified. As a defense mechanism, she taught her body to identify the product that caused the reaction. My patient was neither intolerant nor allergic to adrenaline, because that is physiologically impossible. But she might unconsciously identify the substance if/when it entered her body, thus causing the same reaction she had as a kid. She had developed the most sophisticated and rapid biochemical lab analysis mechanism through connections in her brain. Wow. Talk about a mind-body connection! I learned my lesson.

Chapter 8

Money

I bet some of you jumped directly to this chapter. That's not very smart; for your own good, please return to chapter 1.

This chapter will not be an MBA course on dental economics but will give you some elements that might allow you to understand the basics. Even some dentists who have purchased this book might get their money's worth.

What are the fundamental criteria for of the price you pay for dental treatments? Here is my list, in no particular order:

- Location of the dental practice.
- Appearance of the office. A beautifully decorated, comfortable office requires more investment. That investment needs to be amortized, and you will have to pay for it. But it is more pleasant to walk into a place that shows proof of aesthetics and taste. This counts a lot in dental referrals, although you personally might not look for office appearance when you chose a dental practice.

All I will say, and this is very personal, is that it's not

about the size of the office, the height of the ceilings, or the price of the light fixtures…BUT, if you want a dentist that is detail-oriented and demanding with his or her work, there has to be some proof of it in the way the office is set up, how clean it is, and the effort put into making it delightful and comfortable.

- Staff: Number of people and qualifications.
- Training. The doctor and staff members need training and continuing education. That costs money, sometimes a lot of money. Some advanced, three-day courses for dentists can range between $3,500 and $5,000, plus transportation and accommodations. You will pay higher fees for a more qualified doctor and a well-qualified team. It makes sense.
- Our old friend: Experience! It goes without saying that sometimes experience is overrated – but not in dentistry. Here, the equation is: skill + experience = talent. Experience pays double. You will pay for the extra knowledge it carries.

I would be remiss if I didn't spare a thought for the young dentists who come out of dental school; what should they do, and what should you do? A long, long time ago, I was one of them…. There is no question that for at least the first five years, they must work with someone experienced to shorten their learning curve while under supervision.

What are the advantages of being treated by a junior dentist within a practice of senior colleagues? You, the patient, might get a better fee-for-service without lowering the quality. Yes, you will need to be patient and should not make any other plans on the day of your dental appointment just in case a one-hour consultation turns into four. I hope you know the saying: Cheap, good, and fast is impossible to achieve. You can choose only two of these qualifications for anything you wish to acquire. One of them will have to be sacrificed.

By selecting a young practitioner within an experienced professional framework, you might get the best of both worlds (cheap and good) if you can put in the extra time (the sacrifice). You will also help a young dentist become a skilled professional in the best environment possible. They will remember you forever. Trust me, I know.

- Materials used. To give you an idea, the price of a suitable composite material used for a filling and its adhesive, per gram, is equal to the cost of one gram of gold. Just like in any supermarket, there is an array of brands for most dental products ranging from five-star to generic. Nothing obligates us to buy one or the other, except our ethics, i.e., whether or not we base our purchasing decisions on how much research and development there is behind a product; and the quality of materials we wish to offer.

As in any other field, in the field of dentistry, choose a dentist who *a priori* buys quality products – and no, you cannot tell the doctor what material to use or bring your own! Dental consumables are extremely expensive, sometimes, just because the package says "dental." It's not fair to anyone. Unfortunately, however, you, being the last link in the chain, will pay the price in either money or (lack of) quality.

- A dentist who uses two or three needles to anesthetize a patient. Yes, you will be charged more for the treatments performed, but the price you pay is your well-being.
- The dental lab. This is the unspoken, key link for the entire dental office setup to stand out among the others. Just like the dentist, dental technicians must be highly skilled and well trained. Their dedication is indisputable but not always acknowledged. A lab will have fees, just like us, based on their training, skills, equipment, and experience. The dentist pays those fees. Often, labs must repeat jobs, representing hours of

work and cost in materials, without getting paid, even when the error comes from our end. This will increase the overall cost for the patient because dentists refuse to pay for their re-dos. The math goes wrong when dentists take the lab fee and multiply it by *x* to calculate their fee for a veneer, a crown, or a denture. That practice is okay if they base the quotient on an algorithm of the running costs of the clinic and then apply it to the treatment. But they rarely do. Detailed and real lab expenditure should be specified in the quotation, and invoice, along with an hourly cost for each prosthesis, plus the materials used. Each step in treatment takes us time and consumables, and both can be calculated and added on to the lab fee.

Some European countries are now forcing dentists to specify on patient invoices the actual, real cost of the prosthesis as well as each individual step, in order to force transparency and induce better financial management. Some insurance companies are also asking us to do the same. Along with being fairer to the patient, an added benefit of itemizing costs gives lab techs the recognition they deserve. Yes, dental treatments are expensive and unwelcome, and sometimes arrive when you least expect them, but you must find a way to have the work done instead of postponing or resisting it. Remember, the price can double or triple if you delay. Just think of dental treatment as a commodity. Get a loan from a bank or family members if you don't have the savings, but don't just push it off, unless you accept ending up with a denture for life. Many dental offices will negotiate a loan with their bank for you – yes, at a higher rate – but as we've seen before, 10 percent in interest is much less than a 40 percent rise in overall cost. It is what it is.

Start being dental-smart.

Chapter 9

FAQs

1. What should I look for in the first ten minutes at a dental office?

- Hygiene. Is the place clean? Make sure you use the toilet. If the place is not immaculate, the instruments won't be either. There aren't two standards in one dental office.
- Is the team detail-oriented? Staff members should look neither too sober nor too eccentric. The personality and attitude of the dentist comes out through details such as the overall appearance and presentation of the team as well as their uniforms.
- Observe the other patients in the waiting room. It's not so much about profiling or judging on looks, because a patient base doesn't have to be all that homogeneous, but a doctor who has been practicing for over ten years has patients who reflect unique aspects of her/his personality.
- How do you like the team? What was your first impression of the receptionist, or whoever greeted you? Try asking a simple question, perhaps about whether the practice

offers validated parking. Every member of a team is chosen by the management, so their behavior says a lot about the dentists themselves.

- Do the furnishings and decorative touches stress you out, or does the place give you a relaxed vibe?
- Did a staff member take you into the treatment room (also called an "op")? Did it take the dentist thirty minutes to show up? If so, how was that handled by the rest of the team? Were they too busy running all over the place, or did they show calmness and attention? Did you feel they were available to meet your needs?
- When you met the dentist, did you like the body language? Did he or she smile? How were you greeted? Was the dentist scrolling on a phone screen?

2. Why do I need to go to the dentist every week during treatment? Can this be changed?

There is absolutely no reason for appointments to be weekly. In fact, I have never done this. Some treatments require a healing process between sessions, and that can be anywhere between one week and even six months, depending on the procedure.

Sometimes, if there is lab work, i.e., a dental prosthesis that needs to be made, based on the appliance and the lab, the wait time can range from a few days to a couple of weeks.

I often worked with patients who lived abroad and came only to get a treatment done or something fixed. We would set these patients up for rather lengthy, frequent appointments based on the duration of their stay.

If you must commute interminable distances to go to your dentist, you can request they do as much as possible in each appointment. This has always been my preferred choice. If treatment lasts three months instead of, say, eight, there is less risk of having a patient get demotivated halfway through.

A dentist who sees eight or fewer patients a day will be less stressed out and much more available to meet unpredicted situations which, believe me, will arise. One who sees eighteen patients in the morning and seventeen in the afternoon will be irritated by 2:00 pm because of exhaustion, hunger, and thirst. When you are finished with your treatment for the day and try to book the next appointment, the team will be so proud of the dentist's lack of availability that they might even share their excitement with you: "Sorry, Jane, the doctor can't see you on Monday; she already has seventeen patients." If this is the case, say you will call for an appointment and get out. Busy is good, overbooking is not. Also, a discreet team is a must. Stress exacerbates neurotic behavior, and that cannot be good.

3. In my country, there are specialties in dentistry. When should I go to see a specialist?

The decision to see a specialist is preferably your general dentist's, not yours. Let’s call her a GP, general practitioner. For ease of understanding, I’ll make the specialist a "he." The specialist may have his own practice or could be a member of the same team as your GP.

The advantage of specialists is that they are usually very skilled at what they do. An added plus is that by limiting their field of work, they rapidly gain more experience, and thus expertise. But it is challenging for a specialist, no matter how good he is, to have a global view of a treatment plan, as his focus will be on the treatment he is providing. A well-trained GP will have a view of the journey and the goal, and will coordinate a multidisciplinary case better. When a GP delegates segments of the treatment to a specialist, you want her to be a control freak.

What I think works best is a multidisciplinary team

under one roof. I am a professional control freak, and that has always given me better oversight.

4. How long can I expect a successful dental treatment to last?

That's a tough question to answer. One thing is sure, however: do not stay in a practice that gives you a lifetime warranty. Offering a lifetime warranty in medicine is beyond dishonest and unethical.

The first thing you must remember is that success is dependent during and after treatment on both the dentist and the patient. Responsibility is, in my opinion, 50–50. Here's what you need to do to keep your half of the bargain:

- Rev up your dental hygiene. Hygiene is fundamental. If you have had poor dental hygiene for forty years, and "suddenly" spend a fair amount of money getting your teeth fixed, it will take top-level discipline and will on your part to behave differently. Many of you will not. A tooth with a crown has a higher risk of having a decay than a natural tooth. So does a tooth with a filling. Thus, if brushing is not enhanced after treatment, nothing will last no matter who does it, and no matter how much you pay.
- Please use an electric toothbrush. How

can you buy an iPhone 12 Pro Max with 6 GB of RAM and an A14 bionic processor, and then brush your teeth with a manual tooth-broom, even if it has 150 bristles? Also, please floss unless your electrical brushing is immaculate.

- Wear a nightguard. Wearing this simple appliance is essential to protect the work – and not just for the first four months; forever.
- Go for checkups and cleaning twice a year. This is an absolute must. Throughout my career, the patients who have remained dental-healthy are those who haven't missed a single recall.
- When the dentist sees even a minor cavity, get it done fast. Do not wait.

If you follow these guidelines, the dentist will usually fix anything that goes wrong within the first three years of your treatment, based on your prosthetic/implant warranty. Fillings might not be covered for that long. I call my treatments successes after about eight years, but that's a personal assessment of my work. What I mean by that is that I would like and hope for my dental work to give a minimum of eight years of uneventful comfort. Before you accept a quotation, look at the limited warranty conditions. They are specific to each dental practice. They must seem fair; not too good, not too rigid. Five years on dental is infrequent. Remember: a Boeing 747-8 passenger jet sells for $357 million and comes with only a five-year warranty, even though it's not expected to crash after that time! Generally, planes retire after thirty years of use, but they are constantly checked and maintained. Likewise, your dental work could last ten or twenty years, but it will require maintenance and "repairs."

5. I have had many failed root canal treatments. Isn't it better to extract the tooth and place an implant?

Another tough one. Root canal treatments, classified under the specialty of endodontics, are possibly the most sophisticated treatments aside from some surgical procedures. They require a level of precision and expertise that is impossible to describe to someone who is not a professional.

Two complications can arise from a failing root canal:

a. The root canal looks perfect on an X-ray, and yet, one, two, three years later, it gets infected. The anatomy inside a tooth can be very sneaky; there can be additional nerves, lateral micro tunnels, and whatnot. If all is not entirely well sealed, bacteria will develop.

b. When we do a root canal, we are removing all sources of life from the tooth, including hydration. The tooth becomes brittle starts getting cracks, and the risk of fracture grows exponentially. It will need a crown as soon as possible, but even in that case, a fracture might happen, and the tooth may require an extraction.

In the first case, endodontists who work with a microscope and use 3D radiology to check on the result have a better chance of succeeding. You will pay an arm and a leg for that root canal. Some skilled specialists have top rates of success despite not having such sophisticated equipment, but again, they will be as expensive because of their experience.

In the second case, for all you know, the treatment might have been done by the super-mega specialist from option a, but this might not stop the tooth from fracturing. Then what?

If a tooth fails, you will have the option of a bridge or an implant. When the implant fails, things get even more complicated. I would say, discuss it with the dentist, ask for the warranty policy on root canal therapy as well as the crown that will go over it, and if you can, try to save the tooth.

Run away from dentists who consistently push you to

extract teeth and place implants rather than trying root canals. Generally, their recommendation is based on immediate financial gratification, as perhaps they aren't root canal specialists and dislike referring patients. Alas, this happens way too often. I have placed implants for over twenty-five years. Believe me, they also fail. When in doubt, get another opinion; this isn't marriage.

6. What about periodontal disease or bone disease? Why does this happen, and what can I do about it?

Periodontal disease is a problem that affects the periodontium, which we define as the tissues surrounding the tooth. Surprisingly enough, we know little with regard to why periodontal disease happens, as we haven't been able to link it to a specific gene. We know it's congenital, meaning transmitted from parent to child. We know it's caused by bacteria. It can be aggressive, evolving rapidly. If left untreated, it ultimately causes tooth loss because of the destruction of the supporting bone.

The only factor the patient can control in this scenario is bacteria. Hygiene in a periodontal patient must be extreme. Become obsessive-compulsive with your dental habits if you wish to preserve your oral health and spend your funds on a house rather than your mouth.

This is another reason that you must have regular checkups with the right dentist, because if you are found to have periodontal disease, you will have gotten an early diagnosis. Thus, you can change your behavior in the oral hygiene department before it's too late.

Patients with untreated periodontal disease will lose multiple teeth, and will require implants and, often, grafting techniques to replace the lost bone. Caught early, the disease can be surgically treated. Afterward, the area or the whole mouth will require extensive dental bridgework. Not that many dentists are well trained to do periodontal surgery combined with periodontal prosthetics. You may need to search and visit more than one to find the pearl.

If remained untreated, periodontal disease increases the risk of bacterial migration through the bloodstream. This can cause endocarditis, which is an infection of the tissue that surrounds the heart. Endocarditis is often deadly, so once again, don't underestimate the risks.

7. My husband says that either I'm in love with the female dentist who fixed my teeth or I have Stockholm Syndrome. Is that a thing?

Yes, both can be! The dentist works awfully close to her patients. The recurrent physical contact, added to the fact that we try to make our moves soft and caring, can induce certain feelings, often platonic. The fact that you are a woman, and so is she, does not make it impossible. As for the Stockholm Syndrome, 100 percent yes. In 1973, an escaped convict entered a bank in Stockholm, pulled a gun, and yelled: "The party has just begun!" He kept four people hostage, for over 130 hours. He developed emotional bonds with them, which have since become the stuff of legend and history. Not one hostage spoke severely of him. When he surrendered, the police asked the hostages to come out first, and they refused. They came out with him to prevent the police from shooting him. That relationship is called the Stockholm Syndrome.

I can only wish you all to feel that way once your treatment is over. It will mean you chose well, and you developed the right bond with your dentist.

8. Are dental implants the panacea? Can they fail?

The panacea, if there is one, is keeping your teeth. Nothing will be as perfect as them, nor as well-engineered. Once you lose them, then dental implants become an option. There is no medical solution for anything better than what you had initially. A dental implant is made of titanium, so yes, one enormous advantage is the fact that it does not decay. Aside from that, an implant can develop bone disease, and its treatment is often challenging.

Implants must be checked with X-rays, and more closely than teeth. The moment there is a problem, treatment must be immediate, as the device doesn't have an organic defense mechanism as do teeth. If we don’t check implants regularly and they fail, they can create an extensive bone loss that may very well prevent their replacement. An implant that is failing might not cause discomfort in the first stages; thus, the need for regular checkups.

Implants indeed have the second-highest success rate, right below extractions. Extractions have a 100 percent success rate – you get it, right? Implants in the right hands are at 95 percent. On the opposite end of the spectrum, I have recently seen a so-called dental surgeon with seventeen years of experience have an 80 percent failure rate, destroying mouths and healthy teeth.

Extracting teeth because they are challenging to treat and placing implants instead, is dental mutilation. Alas, many young dentists have been exposed to implants since the beginning of dental school and haven't developed the grit and skills to save teeth like their older, more experienced colleagues. As a result, they often lean toward implantology. Please, do your homework! Your consent to treatment must be well informed and researched. Don't take it lightly.

We now have a website that will allow you to upload X-rays and ask for professional guidance. A team of thoughtful dentists will do their best to help you make the right decision. Find us at www.mental2dental.com.

9. I am upset with my dentist. How should I deal with it?

Your dentist is a human being first and a professional second. Have a discussion; talk to him or her. If you believe we have done something wrong, talk openly. We are not machines, and we can make mistakes. If you think yours is a case of malpractice, or if you can't find a way to have a proper conversation with your dental practitioner, contact your local board of dentists and discuss it with them. They will help you evaluate your case and will mediate with the dentist.

I cannot endorse the conscienceless habit of suing medical professionals, because it's most often motivated by greed. By suing inconsiderately, you are only helping lawyers. It will do nothing for the betterment of our profession or future patients. That's the role of the board of dentists; to regulate how we practice and sanction when required.

Often, another dentist will start criticizing what a colleague has done in your mouth. This is a reason to leave that dentist. An unethical professional will be immoral at all levels. Competent and ethical professionals don't talk badly about other people's work because they know we all can fail. I wish I could reverse this pattern and raise the ethical level of the profession.

I'd also like to raise the moral bar on many patients who seem to be waiting for a well-intentioned doctor to slip up in order to jump on them like a starved lion. How can anyone practice fully and well in such circumstances? After all, they're creating fear for the dentist.

If you want to help create a better world between dentists and their patients, don't listen to lawyers. Lawyers get a cut of what you get. And listen even less to other dentists who push you to sue a colleague.

This proclivity for litigation is a sign of how low we've sunk. Have you ever heard about karma? Make peace, not war.

10. I know smoking is terrible, but I'm addicted to it. I can't imagine the stress of getting my teeth fixed and quitting smoking all at once. What should I do?

My first answer will be a rhetorical question: Where do you think the effects of smoking are felt first? You've got it; in your mouth! It's your body's first filter…but it gets worse.

Do you know that when you take a puff, the temperature inside your mouth is raised to 50° C (122° F)? Considering that the ideal temperature for our cells is 37° C (98.6° F), what do you think the gigantic rise in temperature does to your mouth? No doubt, you can extrapolate that whatever it does, it's not good.

You can try to be smart and say that drinking hot tea is no better, but you aren't inhaling the tea with the agonizing desperation smokers have, as if that puff was the last one they'll ever take! So there goes the smoke with all 7,357 chemicals in it at the speed of a Ferrari, and with the pressure of a tennis ball against your teeth, gums, palate, and cheeks. Right. Maybe you can enjoy it with a gin and tonic!

The direct effect of smoking on the tissues is nasty. The more teeth are missing, the more you are at risk for leucoplakias, which are precancerous lesions in the gums and cheeks. This is because teeth protect the most sensitive tissues from absorbing direct force. The more teeth are missing, the more the smoke, with all it carries, will hit gums and cheeks full on.

I have seen dozens of smokers during my career who came to get implants, and I had to say categorically no, due to the presence of these lesions. While it persists, a leukoplasia should not be disturbed, as more aggression will increase the risk of malignancy. First, the leukoplasia must disappear, then we can consider placing implants. A leukoplasia can quickly turn into oral cancer, which has a survival rate of 50 percent.

Even an extraction on a smoker will heal poorly; you can thus imagine any other type of surgery. With each cigarette, you are destroying collagen, which is one of the vital proteins in the human body. It is the scaffold for all repair processes, bone healing among them. Temperature, chemicals, collagen destruction, oral cancer – even more so combined with alcohol, periodontal disease, bad breath, stained teeth. And we haven't even gone beyond the mouth!

As a dentist, I will fight smokers until my last breath. I have lost too many patients to that stupid, rolled stick of dynamite. To this day, I have yet to perform a bone grafting procedure on a patient who had not quit smoking for at least a month before starting treatment.

So, to answer your question: first, quit smoking and then fix your teeth. Focus your willpower on one thing at a time. You can't expect to succeed at engaging in two willpower-depleting challenges simultaneously. You've waited so long; a month or two won't change your dental situation much. Don't give me an "I want it all, and I want it now." Stop smoking first.

11. As far as I can remember, I have seen my parents wear dentures, and they were happy. Why shouldn't I just go for that if I don't mind having something removable?

Now that is an excellent question. Dentures look good. They look better than any other prosthesis our lab techs can build because everything is artificial in them, both the gum and the teeth. They can look very natural, in which case it's hard for people to know you're wearing one. But there are downsides to dentures, and the younger you begin wearing them, the more the disadvantages will be apparent because you'll need more years from them.

➢ A denture will wear your bone down. The jawbone is right under the gum and gives support to your full dentures. As you wear these, the bone will be resorbed (meaning it will literally progressively disappear), and they will become less comfortable as the years go by. The denture will lose stability and will start moving. This will be even more noticeable on the lower one because you don't have a palate in your lower jaw, and thus, support for this denture is reduced.

- If you have the popular scenario of a full upper denture, lower anterior natural teeth, and a lower posterior partial denture, disaster is guaranteed. This is because your lower anterior natural teeth will hit the front area of the upper denture with so much force that the bone in this area will just crumble. Aesthetics and comfort will deteriorate rapidly.
- Molars are to your chewing muscles as dumbbells are to your biceps. Therefore, the moment you start losing your molars, your biting forces deteriorate as your chewing muscles are no longer stimulated. Patients, and even many dentists, are not aware of this fact. Thus, when we make a denture to replace your molars, the power is no longer there, so you bite harder in order to chew – but you start creating sore spots.

Without your natural molars, by the time you've worn a denture for over five years, you are onto soft food. You think you must replace the acrylic teeth on the denture, not realizing the problem is your muscles. Only posterior implants can bring back your masticatory force.

Your parents' dental expectations were tied to the era in which they lived; they don't have to be yours as well. If you are young, which is as young as you consider yourself to be, and you want comfort for chewing, speech, and aesthetics for as many years as you have to live, it is best to find a compromise between full acrylic dentures and the porcelain fixed solution.

For example, if you have implants placed and an acrylic overdenture made –image below– you get the best of both worlds without the downsides mentioned above. Within the scenario of an acrylic denture over implants, there are different options, which you can find in our Glossary of treatments. If your dentist doesn't offer you the same options available, inquire why, and when in doubt, look for someone who has the right training and thus can offer them.

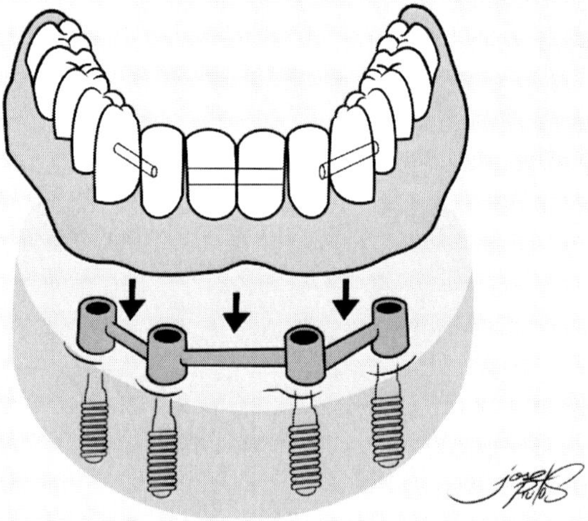

Denture over implants

12. Many years ago, I was given biphosphonates as a treatment for osteoporosis, which I am still taking. I had implants and they all failed. I was told it was due to my condition. Is that true?

Let me start saying a few words about osteoporosis. There is no proven relationship between general osteoporosis and osteoporosis in the jawbones, upper- or lower- maxilla or mandible.

As I mentioned before, activity stimulates bone. There is something called Wolff's law, which states that bone in a healthy person will remodel (modify its structure adapting to the environment) itself to become stronger to resist the load of biting and chewing. Likewise, as you chew, your jawbones are stimulated continuously to withstand the charge – unless you are missing teeth. Whether you are twenty-five or eighty-five, man or woman, you will lose bone density and volume if a tooth is extracted because of the loss of function; again, this is not age-related.

Also, and no matter your age or gender, bone is not the same structurally in the upper or the lower jaws, in the front area or the back. As surgeons, we handle them very differently. Even when we build crowns over implants, we should consider them differently if we want a long-lasting result. In the wrong hands, implants will fail, almost consistently.

As for osteoporosis in the rest of the body, in light of the research I have done – and I am only a dentist – I have come to the conclusion that it is caused by excessive acid in our bodies, and the genius behind our creation provides a mechanism to grab minerals wherever they're available in order to bring the balance back; thus depleting our bones. Minerals from the bones will go into the bloodstream to bring alkalinity back, since that's what they are, alkaline. If we take the problem at the *why* level rather than just medicating ourselves. If we exercise, stop smoking, and modify our food intake to make our body more alkaline, we can reduce the problem considerably. Note that acid foods are not acidic tasting. For example, lemon is one of the most alkaline. I highly recommend you inform yourself and go for a lifestyle change, which will bring health benefits at many other levels.

Now on to bisphosphonates, which is the category of medication you were given.

Just as the pharmaceutical lab Bayer created a precedent by discovering that Aspirin,® an analgesic and anti-inflammatory, could also be used as a blood thinner for patients with some cardiovascular conditions, bisphosphonates, initially designed to treat diseases such as multiple myeloma and metastatic bone cancers, were later found to be helpful in reducing the symptoms of osteoporosis.

Bone is considered an organ with an intrinsic function, which is to sustain the magnificent human body you have. It is the scaffold upon which and within which all is built. As such, it requires constant remodeling. This process is coordinated through complex processes by a group of cells, but we will focus here on only two types: osteoblasts and osteoclasts. The first build bone, the latter destroy it. Simply put, the "clasts" eat the bone and release components that signal the "blasts" to build it anew. Building cannot happen without destruction.

Bisphosphonates impair the process voluntarily,

stopping the destructive action of the osteoclasts. Considering that rebuilding bone takes 150–200 days, bisphosphonates ostensibly allow bone to become stronger.

But there are two downsides to their use. The first is that bone is an incredible material, possessing elastic properties as well as resistance. This combination makes it unique about the way it responds to mechanical stress. It is neither marble nor foam, but a beautifully adaptative component of the human body. If the process of remodeling is medically prohibited, the bone will become stiff and brittle because it will be excessively rigid. Fractures will still happen, and when they do, the repair process is already impaired.

The second drawback is that if there is no remodeling, there is no healing. When we place an implant or do any bone surgery or even a dental extraction, we need osteoclasts for the healing process to start. If they are medically suppressed, patients could get ONJ (osteonecrosis of the jaw, which is the destruction of the bone instead of repair), and implants might fail. Thus, the use of bisphosphonates to systematically and supposedly treat osteoporosis in postmenopausal women prevents them from getting dental implants when they need them the most, after the age of fifty.

If you are taking medication for osteoporosis, tell your dentist immediately so that we can be especially attentive to any healing impairments or complications. Ask your treating doctor about "bisphosphonate holidays," which is a frequent modality for administering biphosphonates. In this case, you are every so often taken off the medication for a certain amount of time, since the effects of the drug remain for several months after you stop.

Do not stop taking the medication on your own or make any treatment decisions without seeking advice from your doctor. He or she will possess the required knowledge, and if not, will consult with someone else. Also, consider changing your diet to include more alkaline food choices; practice sports, including yoga; expose yourself to the sun instead of your TV screen, and don't smoke. You might be pleasantly surprised at the result, and off those meds sooner than you think.

13. What is the ideal dental maintenance, with or without dental restorations?

Let’s go over the main dental maintenance appliances first.

- **An electric toothbrush**. As I emphasized above, using an electric brush is, in my opinion, the way to go. The heads must be replaced approximately every two months. I am not a fan of oral irrigators unless you make sure not to reduce brushing time by using this extra tool.

- **A dental irrigator**. An oral irrigator will give the sensation of cleanliness that ends up making most patients believe it's a good appliance, but it isn't. Nothing can replace the efficiency of a brush.
- **An interdental brush**. See dental irrigators, above. I will say the same for interdental brushes, which are tiny narrow tree shaped ones that fit transversely into the spaces between teeth close to the gum. However, they are indispensable for periodontally affected, as well as implant patients. Likewise, for anyone above the age of forty-five, due to the bone loss, we've naturally suffered. As we lose bone, which is a normal physiological process, small triangles appear between teeth and/or restorations, and they need to be very well maintained. In my opinion, flossing vs. interdental is a no-brainer, the latter wins hands down.
- **Mouthwash**. I believe mouthwashes are way overrated. What's the point? Reason it out yourself: If you need the feeling of freshness, do you really need to put chemicals inside your mouth? Or suppose you want it for disinfection; what is your

mouth, a gutter? What about for wound healing? Well, have you ever heard of the Dead Sea and its miraculous saltwater? That's what we use for healing after surgery, saltwater. Anything else will impair healing, which already says a lot. I have never purchased a mouthwash, nor taken home any of the trillions of samples given to me for free. Next time you get a cut on your finger, try pouring a jet of your mouthwash over it three times a day and watch how the healing goes. Then get back to me.

- **Dental floss**. Oh my. I do have floss at home just in case something gets stuck between my teeth, like chorizo. In fact, the last time I reached for my floss, I found the EarPods I'd lost two months earlier! Granted, the use of floss is indicated with tight contacts or multiple restorations. But ask your dentist or hygienist to teach you how to use it properly. If not, it can do more harm than good.

Each of us must adapt our hygiene methods based on specific anatomical concerns in our mouth, based on the results we have attained so far and on the restorations we have. As you will see in my next book, *Stairway to Implants*, anyone with an implant must always use an interdental brush if they wish to keep the implant healthy. If you have bridges, an irrigator might come in handy – but it's only a plus, not essential. No matter which tools you use above and beyond your two minutes of regular brushing, never replace the toothbrush (or the interdental brushes) with them.

Last, but by no means least, depending on your particular situation, visit a professional every four to six months so they can assess your overall oral health and maintenance habits, as well as clean your teeth and gums comprehensively. If their assessment shows you're doing the right thing, don't change. If anything is wrong, discuss it with the hygienist or dentist and discover what you need to modify so that your results improve. Caring for your teeth requires the mentality of a marathon runner, not a sprinter.

14. In light of the COVID-19 pandemic, I cannot help but wonder what the implications are for dental offices and dental patients. What can you tell me about this?

I was wondering when this question would be asked!

As you may have figured out by now, I don't follow the herd. Granted, I must be compliant with legislation so that my loved ones don't waste time trying to get me out of jail, but that's as far as it goes. For the rest, I keep myself informed by reading well above the average amount my colleagues read, and I draw my own conclusions. In my thirty-five years of practicing dentistry, I don't believe I've ever put a patient's life at risk, nor have I asked my teams to be unnecessarily exposed.

Since the COVID-19 pandemic has become such an overarching part of our lives and will change how we live from now on, it deserves a chapter of its own. See below.

Chapter 10
Dentistry in the Era of COVID-19

I cannot believe I have to write a chapter on what I believe will be written in history books as one of the most significant manipulations ever carried out against humanity.

In my last year of university in the early 1980s, we began to come across cases of unexplained, infectious syndromes that would end up killing their victims. This was the birth of the HIV/AIDS era. It has been and remains a pandemic since Day 1.

The primary means of HIV transmission is unprotected sex, contaminated blood transfusions and hypodermic needles, and mother-to-child during pregnancy, delivery, or breastfeeding. In 2018, 37.9 million people in the world were living with HIV, which resulted in 770,000 deaths in 2018 alone. Close to half of these cases were in East and South Africa. AIDS has caused an estimated 32 million deaths worldwide since the beginning.

In dental practice, we treat every patient as if he or she were an HIV carrier. Why? Because that is the way to protect other patients as well as the staff from cross-contamination.

When HIV appeared, TB (tuberculosis) was slowly disappearing in industrialized countries. However, patients who developed AIDS because they were immunocompromised were more prone to develop TB, which is an opportunistic infection. It gave TB a renewed momentum, and this "old-fashioned" disease came back, more resistant to antibiotics than ever, despite the existence of the BCG vaccine.

Why am I digressing to TB here? Allow me to draw a parallel between TB and COVID-19.

- More than 2 billion people – fully one-third of the world's population – carry a latent form of asymptomatic TB. Ten percent of them can pass it on to others. This means that today, t**wo billion** people will test positive for Mycobacterium tuberculosis, the bacteria responsible for TB. They can develop the disease at any point in time if their immune system weakens – and likewise transmit it.
- Worldwide, there are 8.4 million new tuberculosis cases a year. Every single day: winter, spring, summer, or fall, 4,100 people die of TB.
- People with HIV are thirty times more likely to develop TB. Infants and young children are more susceptible to contracting severe forms of TB, such as meningitis.

➢ People with diabetes are three times more likely to develop TB.

➢ People in dusty environments and the mining industry are at increased risk of developing TB. Their lungs present the same patterns doctors are using to label hospital patients as "COVID-diseased."

- Note that mines are a ubiquitous part of the landscape in northern Italy.
- Note that China and Italy[8] are the world's largest producers of ceramic by far, and respiratory health problems among ceramic workers are well-documented.
- Smokers are at higher risk of developing TB and any other respiratory disease. Thirty percent of the cigarettes in the world are consumed in China – which comprises 18 percent of the world population.
- The gender breakdown for smokers is 40 percent of men and 9 percent of women.
- TB is transmitted by the saliva; micro-droplets are projected when coughing, sneezing, and speaking.

---

[8] The Canadian Mineralogist43(3):935-950 DOI: 10.2113/gscanmin.43.3.935 Giorgio Garuti FedericaZaccarini

Now, have you ever heard of social distancing with TB? Have you ever seen, anywhere, the obligation to wear masks to prevent TB contagion?

Have you ever seen a dentist work two meters away from you, or wear a spacesuit to treat you in case you were one of those 2 billion TB carriers?

I'm giving you this data to make you think; I'm not telling you what to think. I have my opinion, and that's all it is. Try to understand and draw your own conclusions, but not by watching the news on TV. There, you are already swallowing the findings others are force-feeding you as if you were a goose being fattened for foie gras. We are not animals. We do not belong to a herd, a flock, or a swarm. If you were meant to be one, you wouldn't be reading this. We have a mind, and free will, and if you don't exercise them, why be here at all?

Here are the numbers: In 2018, an estimated 10 million people fell ill with tuberculosis (TB) worldwide. 5.7 million men, 3.2 million women and 1.1 million children[9]. There were cases in all countries and age groups.

Twenty-five out of one hundred people in the world –

---

[9] Information from who.int website published in March 2020

one out of four – are carriers of the TB bacterium. Ten percent of these individuals are contagious even without symptoms. That is 2.5 percent of the world population. It means that 2–3 out of 100 patients in a dental office can transmit the TB bacterium to others.

Let's look at the testing Iceland has conducted so far on COVID-19 (which is the only one that makes sense to me). They have tested 13 percent of their population *randomly*; fifty thousand people in total, and *not in hospitals*. Hospital testing is already biased.

Fewer than one percent tested positive for the virus. Fifty percent of them were asymptomatic, meaning they could spread the virus, though less effectively than ill patients. So out of one hundred people, we can assume that less than one will test positive for the coronavirus and let us say that one out of two hundred can transmit the disease without being sick.

It appears that a major difference between COVID-19 and TB is that healthy people with the coronavirus *can* transmit it in its active form, but less efficiently than an ill patient. This means that the sick person is more "dangerous" than a non-sick carrier, thus making protection much easier than with silent TB. Well, allow me to say that there is another major difference between Covid-19 and TB. Covid-19 is killing in western countries more than third world nations. Aha. Of course.

TB didn't merit being all over the news on World Tuberculosis Day 2020, which was on March 24th. Why?

For one, more people die of TB in underdeveloped countries, so the fact that you can own a Tesla and be the CEO of a company and still die from COVID-19 makes it more dramatic than TB. *Really*? Yes. We are not all born equal.

But COVID-19 is here to put things back into perspective and prove that we are.

Tuberculosis is old news. Furthermore, there's already a vaccine against it, which means no patent potential for millionaire wannabes.

COVID-19 is also about fear. Fear creates separation, and fear suppresses the immune system. Throughout history, you can see how fear has been used to manipulate masses and commit the biggest crimes against humanity! Medical fear can be put in a separate category from other types of fear because it remains hidden behind a screen of respectability. That must change. What belongs to the medical field is not necessarily respectable. In the medical field, there is also huge financial interest at the corporate and individual levels, and big egos are involved. Just because you have the initials of an international organization, don't believe it is true. They also need money and have huge salaries and trips to pay. A book on fear could be written based on COVID-19 alone. All we can do now is wait and see who makes the biggest amount of money on this episode. There you will find some of the manipulators. Others will remain hidden for now.

Bringing it back to the dental office, let's assume that I'm a carrier of either TB or COVID-19 and can transmit it to you. How? By sneezing right on your face? Or by carrying it on my clothes? What if you are a carrier? If your clothes are infected, you'll pass the bacteria or virus on to my clothes and the dental chair, which, in any case, always has to be disinfected between patients – remember we discussed the importance of cleanliness in a dental office?

What does make sense, more than the doctor wearing a spacesuit that will make our work highly tricky, is having the patient, doctor, and nurse all wear a single-use gown – which is what we already do during implant or grafting surgery. We can also don single-use headwear and shoe protectors to simplify our disinfection procedure, and that's it. For the rest, a clinic that has always been clean will be fine. But beware and look for signs of cleanliness.

I have been in many, many dental clinics in my life. I have seen things I cannot describe here, as I am trying to motivate you to get on with your treatment! And I will always look at the good that comes out of every situation. Happily, coronavirus has forced medical offices to put single-use plastic on treatment chairs and equipment. For me, it's not about COVID-19. I've been obsessive-compulsive all my life in my work environment, but believe me, not all dentists are. There are scary bacteria that live in a dental clinic, and you might be carrying some on your clothes as well. Consequently, this return to creating a sterile medical environment is a good thing.

It's not about living in a germ-free environment; I'm not like that. I lived in Africa and brushed my teeth with tap water! But dental offices require a level of cleanliness that is impossible to achieve at the rate we see patients nowadays – and given the lack of consciousness, there was until now. Fear and paranoia aside, this is a perfect time to permanently embrace the changes COVID-19 has brought. You probably know these changes will come at a price. The equipment now required has a cost-per-patient-treated tag. What's more, the time required to prepare treatment rooms is going to be affected, lowering the productivity of the office and thus raising the overhead. But hey, it is what it is. Everything happens for a reason. Look at the positive outcomes and let go of the rest. Resistance is useless and only works against you.

Equipment and instrument sterilization techniques must always be on an HIV, hepatitis, and TB obsessive-compulsive standard, so again: verify the cleanliness of the office by looking at simple details.[10] Please try not to be afraid of the new post-COVID-19 reality. All it will do is increase your risk of not wanting to visit us, thus making your treatment more complex and expensive as time goes by. Be logical and think. Stress and fear paralyze all of us. You don't need a PhD to understand how it works. The most reluctant patients will use COVID-19 as an excuse for dental laziness. Laziness is an obstacle to fearlessness. So beware

---

[10] See the beginning of chapter 9 for more information on what to look for in a dental office.

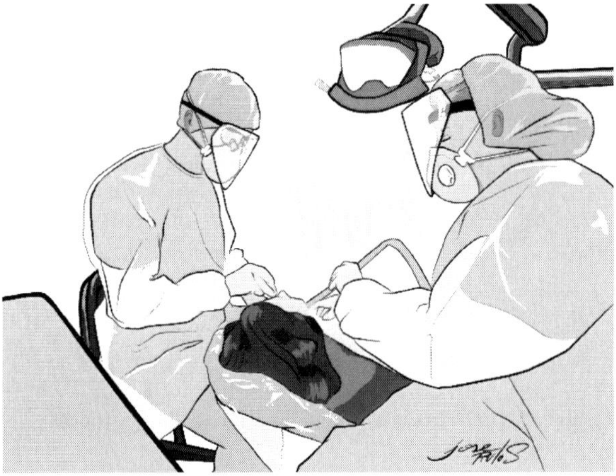

CONCLUSION

"The price is high; the reward is great."

—Maya Angelou

For the Dentist

After thirty-five successful years in the dental profession, I have drawn many conclusions, some of which appear in this book. The one thing I'm completely sure of is how much my patients have helped me grow. They have helped me overcome dramas that shook my life, sometimes through their mere presence and sometimes through their advice. Of course, they have helped me make an excellent living and bring up my daughter as a single mother. More fundamentally, however, my patients sparked my initial wonder of and fascination with human nature. Through their stories and challenges, I was able to better understand the human equation.

My ability to focus has always been such that I could do the technical work fast and well – which gave me plenty of time to chat with patients. Many became friends and would often say I was their psychologist. To me, this is fifty percent of the job.

As we all have seen in our own practice, beliefs inform the way a person perceives pain. If patients know we love and care for them, they will not expect pain. Their journey under our care will be one of a person going to see a friend who will be taking care of their problem together with them. When or if something does not turn out as expected, they will not get upset; the two of you will discuss it and will together do your best to find a solution. Thus, a challenge will not become a drama because the patient relates to us as a human *being* and not only a human *doing*.

This is why psychology is more than half of what we do. We need psychology every second we practice dentistry. It is not possible to be friends with all our patients, but it is possible to be at peace with each of them. And if you do find yourself with a patient you cannot even be at peace with (and vice versa), I advise you, as the doctor, to terminate the relationship before it sours irreparably. For both your sakes, suggest the patient look for another dentist. Yes, patients, we do have the right to do so, but we will not leave you stranded in the middle of the road. We do have an obligation to finish our cases, but what will be the end result if we are both uncomfortable with each other and can't seem to get along?

That being said, and because we are human, we must also own our mistakes and embrace our vulnerability. Right before COVID-19 kicked in, I was hired to help a team of dentists in a poorly managed, huge dental practice. The pile of complaints on my desk was humongous. I had never personally been hit with a lawsuit in my life, not even a mean claim, and here I was working at a clinic that had been functioning for only three years and dealing with more disasters than I could handle.

Once, as I was taking leave of a patient after a long meeting trying to find a solution to their mess, I apologized and warmly accompanied them to the door. My boss said to me, "We should never apologize. We should not acknowledge we have done something wrong, because they will sue us."

I then understood where their problem was coming from and why I wouldn't be able to help them. The whole company culture was backward. The need for control and the arrogance behind it will ignite even the most innocent patient – now *that's* an oxymoron.

So yes, be humble; you owe it to your patients. You are not God. Your patients have chosen you. That should awaken gratitude and humility, not arrogance. Be grateful, be empathetic and compassionate. After that foundation is laid, you can prove how good a dentist you are.

Most dental schools don't teach more than twenty hours of psychology during the six-plus years of graduate training. It is what it is. But if you are committed to learning and improving, believe me, the rest will follow. Humility and empathy will also hold your team together, including members of the dental lab. We are neither solo players nor the stars of the show, even though we may think we are. Without our assistants, hygienists, front desk team, practice manager, lab techs, and any other support staff in our office, we are nothing. So think of them first and stop using them as escape valves. Run 10K every morning if you need to, but respect your team as you respect your family. We try so hard not to hurt patients, but sometimes we hurt the people who work with us and help us be the best every day.

For the Patient

The two most important ingredients for successful dental care are **courage** and **awareness**. Let's tackle them separately.

I'd like to put the topic of money aside for a moment, and stuff fear and doubt into a bottle. Okay, now that we've taken care of money and fear, what do you need to overcome whatever has been preventing you from going to the dentist? Courage, nothing more. Courage is not the absence of fear. Courage is knowing what you need to do to become the person you wish to become. Courage is letting go of all the excuses anchored in your past experiences. Courage is facing your current situation, embracing it and then, stepping up. Courage is not complaining about your current situation, while visualizing where you want to be as far as oral health is concerned. Courage is finally, making the right financial decisions to be able to move forward.

Fear is a small player based on uncertainty and projection. Most of the things we are afraid of will never happen anyway. Hold on to your courage; it is a gift we all have. Choose to step up, and you'll be okay.

Now onto awareness. Oral care is not about slapping a credit card on the receptionist's counter and showing the dentist your teeth. It's about having an awareness of what we have done for you, of the care we have taken to respect your human dignity by providing you with the best dental treatment we can possibly give you, and of the efforts that a team of professionals has made to get you to your goal.

No doubt the above paragraph has caused some of you

to stir upon your chair indignantly. "What you've done for *me*? I paid you an arm and a leg!" Go back to the beginning of the book. It's not about what you've paid. The efforts real dental professionals make cannot be given a price tag. Dentistry is a profession that affects our nerves, our hearing, our back, and our personal lives more than any other. Yes, we get paid, but I'm talking about the value and quality we bring to your life with what we do.

It is my hope that you will remember these two things when you are done reading: the courage it took for you to step up, and an awareness of the value you received.

***

When Maya Angelou said, "The price is high; the reward is great," she wasn't talking about money, and neither am I. This is true for every single one of us in this fantastic, epic, love-hate relationship between dentists and their patients which gives birth to so many comic anecdotes, humorous videos, and horror stories.

Every body – spelled intentionally with two words – needs a dentist to care for it, and every dentist needs patients in order to grow and survive. It takes both to succeed.

GLOSSARY OF TREATMENTS

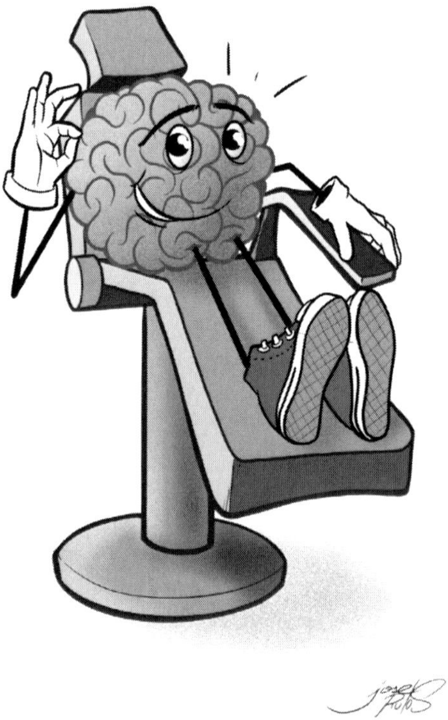

The following treatments, and others not mentioned here, can comprise a *Treatment Plan* (TP). The TP a dentist gives you is as important as what an architect will present to you before building your dream house. Some of what is written here has been covered briefly in chapter 9, but in this Glossary, I will go into greater depth.

To design a suitable TP, we must look at the whole mouth, not just the tooth you keep pointing at. When you go to the ophthalmologist, you allowing him or her to examine both eyes even if you feel pain only in the right one. However, when it comes to your mouth, if you point to the upper right, if we even turn our head toward your left side, you hold our hand like Mr. Bean and immediately say, "No, no, this one!"

The mouth is an organ, and as such, we need to examine it thoroughly and repair whatever we see is wrong in it. Anything else is malpractice. If your dentist examines only the tooth that hurts you, change dentists.

Crowns and Bridges

A crown is a prosthetic reconstruction that covers a tooth. It can serve one of two purposes. One is to reinforce a weakened tooth, usually after a root canal.

(Just to remind you, if you have not had root canal in that tooth, the treatment of choice is an onlay.) A premolar or molar with a root canal should always and immediately get a crown. If you wait, you will lose the tooth. The other purpose of a crown is to cover a living tooth when it is used as part of a bridge.

A bridge is made to replace one or more missing teeth, using remaining natural teeth as support. It is the alternative to implants, and vice versa. When a bridge is made over vital teeth – teeth that still contain the nerve – the practitioner must ensure not cause irreversible damage to the pulp (nerve). There is still a chance that the tooth could still require endodontic (root canal) treatment later; it's one of the reasons why implants can be a better option.

Crowns and bridges can be made from metal-ceramic or zirconia-ceramic. A metal-ceramic bridge or crown doesn't imply that the metal will be visible, but it will require a more skilled ceramist–lab tech. The ceramic covers the metal, and in my opinion, is still the treatment of choice today, as metal gives a better seal at the margins.

Nevertheless, most reconstructions are made with zirconia, as the digital era has brought with it machines that mill zirconia. Often, at least for single crowns, the dentist will have the milling machine in-house and will make your crown on the go. This arrangement works for posterior teeth, but the naturalness and transparency of a beautiful front tooth demands an artist-ceramist lab tech to build the aesthetic layer on top of the zirconia.

Dentures

Acrylic partial denture

An acrylic removable partial denture, should not be considered a final restoration, as you will lose your remaining teeth and end up with a full denture! Acrylic partial dentures are temporary appliances only.

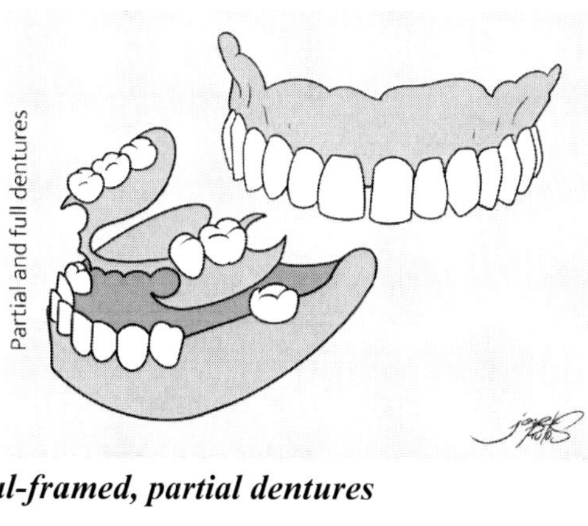

Metal-framed, partial dentures

This is the right option if you must wear a removable denture because of financial issues or lack of bone for implant placement. Your remaining teeth must be appropriately restored and prepared for the denture, and in the right hands, it will give you comfort and a durable solution.

Full denture

This is the option when you have no teeth left, as well as no money or no bone for implants. A full denture is removable and will give you good aesthetics and better comfort, especially for the upper jaw. It should be removed at night and seen/fixed by a dentist or denturologist once a year – depending on the law in your country[11]. As you continually keep losing bone, it should be refilled so that it fits accurately and remains stable. In that way, you will reduce further bone loss. If you can wear implants, there are different options for combining them with dentures that can give you a much better quality of life. Please refer to our implant guide below for more details.

---

[11] Some countries such as Canada or Australia, allow for lab technicians to see patients, make, and adjust removable dentures directly without the need for the patient to see a dentist. They are called denturologists.

Fillings

A filling is the most conservative dental restoration. It is done when a decay/cavity is present on a tooth. It is made by the dentist in one go, with **composite-resin** (white) or **amalgam** (gray). Despite the long-term crusade against amalgam fillings initiated in 1841 by the American Society of Dental Surgeons and perpetuated by the World Health Organization (WHO), amalgam fillings are the most durable and mechanically resistant material that has been made to this date.

The United States Food and Drug Administration, the World Dental Federation, the Mayo Clinic, the American Cancer Society, the American Academy of Toxicology, the Environmental Protection Agency, and even WHO had to acknowledge that amalgam fillings lasted longer than any other material and presented no health risk for patients. Yet WHO is still promoting the phasedown of dental amalgam in developing countries, which are the ones that can least afford treatment failure. At this time, they are using the excuse of environmental consequences in underdeveloped countries, as well as the effects of cremating bodies that contain amalgam. Really? What volume of amalgam does this realistically represent?

I have amalgam fillings. Most dentists stay away from composite materials for themselves, mainly because resins shrink as they set, thus leaving a gap for bacteria to grow from the moment they are made.

It is essential to know that any restored tooth will always be at a higher risk of getting decayed than a healthy tooth, no matter the material. This is due to the junction that exists between the tooth and the restoration, which inevitably will always have a gap. Moreover, there are often areas we seal blindly as we have no visual access to them. This becomes more critical with composites because they shrink as they harden, thus creating a separation between the material and the tooth. Why do we do them, then? Because of patients' demand for aesthetics.

The best alternative to an amalgam filling is a porcelain **onlay** (see below). If you want aesthetics, you have to pay for it. If you can't afford to get an onlay, then settle for an amalgam filling that will last an average of fifteen years.

Gingivectomy

A gingivectomy is a procedure performed on the gums to improve the aesthetic result of an anterior restoration

or to gain access to the healthy tooth structure to save a deeply decayed tooth. To put it bluntly, we cut the gum to give a new contour. As we have seen in chapter 5, in an aesthetically oriented dental practice, gingivectomy will often be combined with veneers or anterior crowns. Anterior implant cases may also require gingivectomy, as the gum level on implants is not easily predictable but can always be corrected.
The best tool for performing gingivectomies with regard to result and postoperative comfort is a soft-tissue laser,

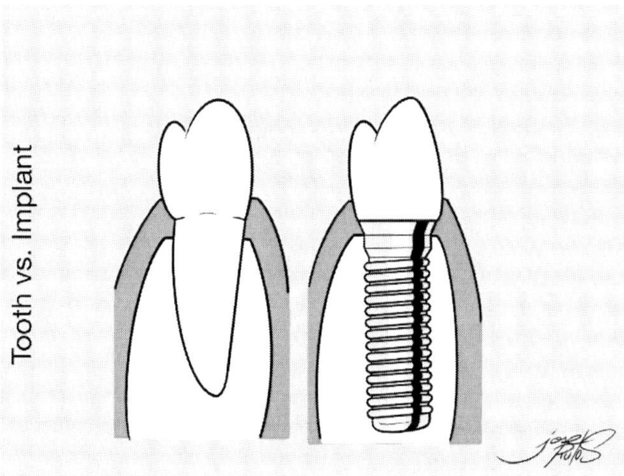

available in most practices nowadays. Make sure your dentist has it.

Implants and Bone Grafting

A natural tooth comprises the outside part you see, which we can call *the clinical crown*, and the root – one or multiple – which is inside the jaw, surrounded by bone. When a tooth is extracted, we remove it all. Dental implants are titanium fixtures we insert inside the bone to mimic the role your original root was playing.

An implant is a screw-like element that replaces the root. After this procedure, a crown will be made to replace the clinical crown. Thus, a tooth can be replaced with a bridge or an implant. As we've learned above, in most cases a bridge implies damage to healthy teeth, whereas implants are standalone units that do not require the support of healthy teeth. In fact, implants and teeth should never be connected.

Immediate implants

Immediate implants are placed at the time of extraction. Many dentists perform them as a matter of course, but they are a double-edged sword. Make sure you are the one in a hurry, not the dentist, and make sure you understand the repercussions if the implant fails. It requires a highly skilled and experienced surgeon to place immediate implants successfully. It also requires a set of prerequisites. If one of them is not met, it is always safer to delay the implant placement. Make sure you ask for both the pros and cons of immediate implants, and *you* make an informed decision.

Delayed implants

These are the most common implants. Generally, tooth extraction and implant placement are at least eight to twelve weeks apart. This allows for the bone to fill the gap left by the extraction and the implant to be placed in the ideal conditions in healthy bone.

Waiting longer to place the implant is not a problem, although waiting for more than a year can cause bone loss. As I said in chapter 9: What allows for the bone in your jaws to be maintained is the stimulation generated initially by your dental root and later by the dental implant. In the absence of a structure inside the bone, you will lose volume irreversibly. Therefore, if you wait for too long to have the money, you will not have any bone left, and will need a bone graft!

Bone grafting

Bone grafting may be needed if you have lost bone, due to either disease, the extraction itself, or time. The most efficient bone grafts to increase the thickness will be autologous, meaning we take your bone from somewhere else in your mouth to recover the required anatomy. We can take bone from inside your mouth, or from around the knee, the hip, or the skull.

Sinus elevations are a specific type of bone graft that,

based on your anatomy, are sometimes needed in order to place implants in the molar region. In the right hands, they have a low rate of complications. Sinus elevations do not require autologous bone unless a large amount of grafting is required.

There is too much information about implants and bone grafts to share here. Look out for my next book, *Stairway to Implants*.

Nightguards

Nightguards are usually transparent, acrylic-based appliances worn on one arch alone (only upper or lower jaw). Patients wear them at night to protect their natural teeth and/or the restorative work achieved during dental treatment. If they are made to fit tightly on your teeth, they will play an essential role in stopping teeth from further movement. An example of this would be a night guard worn after orthodontic treatment to maintain the attained result. Another reason to wear a nightguard is to prevent more chaos when teeth are already crooked.

There are two types of night guards. The most frequent is thick, full-arch nightguard made of soft material. In my opinion, this type enables you to chew all night and can cause muscle discomfort. The second type of night guard is the one developed by Dr. Gene McCoy. It is rigid; usually, 1.5 mm thick, and will generally span from canine to canine, if the bite is normal and canines are healthy. By decreasing contacts between posterior teeth, the biting forces developed at night are lessened, thus allowing for muscle relaxation and preventing overstimulation of the chewing muscles.

The rigid night guard is less frequently used because of habit. Labs usually make them out of soft silicone, and since there is no real training on the topic, it became the trend. Therefore, you must make sure that you request a rigid partial night guard. Don't hesitate to refer to our website www.mental2dental.com for more information on this. Innumerable patients have thanked me and praised the rigid night guard once I started delivering them. It's also the one I've personally used on myself for over twenty years. As a grinder, having broken teeth and having had severe TMJ (temporomandibular joint) issues, I cannot recommend this type of night guard enough.

Onlays

An onlay (or inlay; they differ in shape) is a gold or porcelain filling-like restoration made by the dental lab. It is better than a filling for this exact reason. As it is made by the lab on a stone model, which in turn is based on a silicone or digital impression, all margins (junction between the tooth and the lab restoration) are accessible to the lab tech's eye. Consequently, and onlay is made with much higher precision, thus guaranteeing a better prognosis for its life span.

Onlays cost more but consider the following scenario. You need a tooth treated. It's too damaged to safely give it a filling, but not compromised enough to require a root canal. Nevertheless, you still request a filling to save money. The tooth will end up needing a root canal, a post, and a crown; or an extraction. That is the only thing guaranteed. In the end, it will cost you a lot more money.

Many dentists will offer a crown rather than an onlay. Why? Crowns and onlays often cost the same for both you and us, but the onlay is more technique-sensitive, thus requiring more training. It also requires more time for the dentist and the lab. The only way the profession will go toward the more conservative onlays instead of crowns (assuming they're indicated in the specific case) is if they are a bit more expensive to the patient.

Once again, if you can afford it and the tooth does not have a root canal, do an onlay to preserve the integrity of the organ. And note that not all dentists know how to do onlays. This is the raw reality. Find a dentist who gives you the option. It will mean he or she knows how to do them.

Oh, yes, gold or porcelain? Dentists will say gold hands down. I know you must be thinking I'm at least eighty-five years old and belong to the era of the cave-dentist. Seriously, though, in Europe, the standard of care is the yellow gold onlay for restoring posterior teeth that don't require root canal treatment. That's what most well-trained dentists will get for themselves if they need a tooth filled, and for the patients who can make the right choice—just saying.

Post and Core Reconstruction

A post and core reconstruction is made either by the dentist or by a lab tech. The goal is to replace the part of the tooth that was destroyed by dental disease, as well as whatever had to be removed to perform the root canal. If there is enough dental structure left, it can be done by the dentist in one go with a fiber post, which reduces the risk of tooth fracture.

If the tooth remnant is too weak, however, then the post and core will be made out of metal by the lab. In this case, the dentist's skills are more critical, as the risk of fracture increases due to the biomechanical differences between metal and the tooth. Either way, the post and core will sit under the crown. And in some specific cases, when working with metal, the post and the crown can also be one piece.

Root Canal Therapy (endodontic treatment)

A root canal is needed when a cavity has reached the nerve (also called the pulp) or is too close to it for a filling or onlay to be done successfully. It consists of removing the nerve and replacing it with a medication that stays inside the root permanently. A successful root canal is one where the medicated paste completely fills the contour of the root, and it must be dense enough to prevent bacteria from growing within tiny existing voids[12]. It is a technically challenging procedure, and even when it looks perfect on an X-ray, it often gets infected. That being said, the root canal should always be tried. If you

---

[12] Alas, even in what seems to be on an -ray a successful looking root canal there are often tiny existing voids where bacteria can be lodged.

can afford a specialist, it's even better.

A root canal can fail up to fifty percent of the time. As a result, there is a trend to extract teeth and place implants based on statistics, because implantology has a 95 percent success rate, *in the right hands.* I cannot emphasize enough that you should always try to save teeth. Implants will not last a lifetime unless lifetime is short.

Note that, more often than not, a tooth that has had endodontic treatment will need a crown placed on it due to the increased risk of the treated tooth fracturing. It will also require a post-reconstruction (refer to the section above on post reconstruction).

Temporaries

Temporaries are usually acrylic (resin) crowns, bridges, or dentures that are meant to be worn – yes, you guessed it – temporarily, either while the lab is making your final reconstruction or while you are undergoing healing processes between treatment sessions. If they are removable appliances, they should be worn as little as possible so that healing is undisturbed. When they are fixed, care should be given to the food you eat, as they will easily break if you chew nuts or open beer bottles with them.

Temporaries should be aesthetically and functionally acceptable even though they are going to be replaced by the permanent appliance. And yes, you should judge the professional by the temporaries you get. If your dentist focuses on making them beautiful, it shows how much attention they will pay to their final work. Don't think that because it is temporary, it doesn't matter.

Veneers

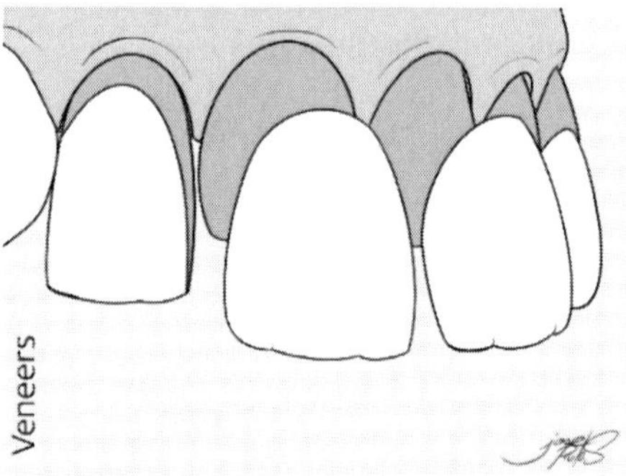

Veneers are thin laminates – usually made of porcelain because it's the most aesthetic material – and placed on the surface of anterior teeth to correct defects in color, shape, or mild position. The dental lab makes the veneers; therefore, treatment requires at least two appointments. The space occupied by the veneer will have the corresponding amount of enamel removed on your tooth to account for the thickness of the restoration, thus making it the right volume.

While the Veneer is being made, you will have to wear a temporary that could sometimes be as temporary as the time it gets you to go back to your car. Oh well, as Buddhists say, all is impermanent.

In the right hands, veneers are one of the most successful restorative treatments, and much less invasive than crowns. Though you may end up needing a root canal because of the anatomy or the position of the tooth, the chances this will happen are lesser than with a crown. Even if you do end up needing a root canal, the risk of the tooth fracturing in the future is less than with a crown, because overall, we have removed less substance. (Remember that you should never choose a crown if the problem is discoloration, shape, or a mild position defect.)

Whitening

Contrary to popular belief, having your teeth whitened by a professional does not damage them. What we do in a dental office is not comparable to anything you can buy over the counter and off the shelf. We use concentrations and specialized products that are much more efficient. We also use ultraviolet light or laser to activate the product, which enhances its whitening potential. If you want full-on efficiency, a professional whitening always has to be followed by at-home bleaching with custom-made bleaching trays for at least two weeks. The reason for this is that the slight reversible alteration of the enamel caused by the product we use in the office will remain for about fifteen days. Therefore, not only can you enhance the result by using a whitening product for as long as the enamel "pores" remain open – it's a metaphor, but close to reality – you can also avoid immediate staining when the enamel is the most prone to it.

It is also of utmost importance during these fifteen days to avoid drinking colored carbonated sodas – which you should avoid anyway at all times since they also lower your saliva's Ph. Stay away from any foods made with strong coloring agents, such as saffron, turmeric, and even cinnamon. No oranges or their juice, tea, or coffee, red wine, or any other colored drinks. If you have an addiction to any of these, and do not want to desist from consuming it, brush your teeth right after drinking. And Do Not Smoke!

THE END

LIST OF CONTRIBUTORS

Thanks to José Rulos for his amazing illustrations and cover

Thanks to Deena Nataf for the wonderful work done editing this manuscript

INDEX

Dear Reader,

Thank you for reading my book – I'd love to hear about your thoughts and reactions.
You can **write to me** on our website

https://mental2dental.com/c-k-labalen/

You must know how important reviews are for us, So please can I kindly ask you to leave a review to help others benefit from this read? Make it your way of paying it forward □. Thanks. Namaste

LOG IN TO YOUR AMAZON ACCOUNT, GO TO THE PAGE WHERE YOU PURCHASED THE BOOK, SCROLL ALL THE WAY DOWN , AND CLICK ON WRITE A REVIEW….PLEASE. GOOD OR BAD, IT IS IMPORTANT.

Made in United States
North Haven, CT
20 October 2026

20740140R00099